# Your Health in Your Hands

Dr Smita Naram

Copyright © 2016 Dr Smita Naram

The right of Dr Smita Naram to be identified as the author of this book has been asserted.

A CIP catalogue record for this book is available from the British Library.

Published by Ayushakti Health Publications

ISBN 978-90-822141-0-9

With thanks to

Persia West

for interviewing, editing, writing

and bringing this book together

**Local contacts for Ayushakti clinics, and for products referred to in the text**

**India**

www.ayushakti.com

**1800 266 3001**

**USA**

www.ayushaktiusa.com

1800 280 0906

**Germany**

www. Ayushakti.de

49 89 347300

**Europe/UK**

www.ayushakti.eu

0031 181 614017

**Australia/New Zealand**

www.ayushakti.au

# Contents

# My Story

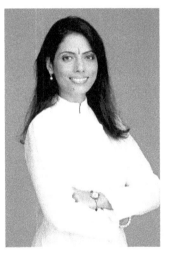

Ayurveda is in my blood. My grandfather, my great—grandfather, in fact going back four generations on my father's side, were all Ayurvedic doctors. For that reason, from my earliest childhood, my father gave me Ayurvedic herbs for my health rather than using chemical—based medicine.

I clearly remember one incident, a striking example from when I was 10 years old, which demonstrated to me the effectiveness of using Ayurveda. I had severe colic, which was very, very intense. I was rolling round on the floor in pain, screaming; I thought I was going to die. My father took me to see a physician, who said it might well be appendicitis and they may have to operate. We'll wait for a day, even half a day, he said, and if it doesn't go away, we'll operate. This was around 1972, when there was no sophisticated diagnostic machinery as there is now. People didn't think clearly; they just thought—this is appendicitis, so we'll operate if there's pain and that will end the problem. That was it.

We went back home and my father called on my uncle, who was a very famous Ayurvedic doctor in our village in Gujarat. My uncle the doctor, when he heard the diagnosis and solution, said, 'No, no, there's no need for surgery; we'll just give her an enema. 'So he gave us a formula we could make from what we had in the house; a mixture of cumin, dried ginger powder, ajwain, asafoetida, coriander and other things, which we boiled and added to castor oil in specific quantities. My father then gave me an enema of this mixture. Within five minutes I cleared my bowels completely, released lots of gas, and with this the pain disappeared. This was my foundation experience of the effectiveness of Ayurveda.

Then, when I was just fifteen years old I met Dr Pankaj Naram, at a spiritual organisation which taught the principles of The Bhagavad Gita. Pankaj inspired me to study Ayurveda, which he was already deeply into. So I started studying Ayurveda, and completed my formal studies by 1981.

I then thought it would be good to study pharmacy, in order that we could then make our own high quality products. So I did a full-time three year pharmacy course, and also did part-time business management and admin. By 1986 I had started full-time Ayurvedic practice.

So that's how my journey started. While I was still studying, and Pankaj was teaching me pulse-reading in the evenings; I would study in the day and every evening I would go to the clinic where he was practicing. I learned pulse-reading for about three years, constantly learning, up until 1985.

All of my training was directly under Pankaj, but actually he never formally trained anybody. He always said that you must observe, observe, observe and observe the pulse. He gave some basic guidelines and then I was observing constantly. By that process I became very refined in my ability.

Finally, after five years of practice, I became extremely good at pulse reading, and practised it side by side with my pharmacy experience, adding further training with another teacher Vaidhya Bhave to gain knowledge on Panchkarma, Ayurvedic detoxification.

When I first began feeling the pulse, all I could detect was that this person was alive, the heart was beating. Then, gradually, after seeing 80 to 100 people every day, new insights began to arise, and I began to know where toxins were located, for example in the upper or lower part of the body, or the digestive tract, as well as the nature of the toxin, whether it was hot or cold, or mixed with air. From this I began to be able to understand what was going on within a patient more deeply. I could see, for example, that people who had hot toxins in the head would normally suffer from headaches and anger, with skin problems on the scalp.

If through the pulse I found mucousy cold toxins in the head region, along with low immunity levels, people would definitely suffer from allergies, sinusitis, coughs and colds. Using the pulse in this way I could recognise a whole range of issues, such as fibroids, polycystic ovary syndrome, male infertility, tube blockages, arthritis, auto immune problems, the location of pain and the reasons for either inflammation or degeneration, allergies, migraines, blood pressure, diabetes; a whole range of health issues. This helped to define the process behind the symptoms; the hidden factors behind what we can see, then precisely focusing on these hidden influences and remove them, so that symptoms vanish naturally.

I also spent a lot of time developing herbal formulas, because I saw that the classical Ayurvedic formulas had many shortcomings in our modern age. When these formulas were created, two or three thousand years ago, the culture was more Kapha than now.

This means that people were more tranquil, quieter, life was easy, it wasn't so fast-paced. The way of living was slow. If you had to travel it took a long time. If you travel in a fast vehicle as we now do, it increases Vata, but that was not a problem in those days. A long time ago people travelled in Kaphic vehicles—such as ox carts—

which did not increase Vata. Stress levels were not high; the diseases of that time were more Kapha-related. So when we looked at their formulas we found they used lots of herbs for increasing heat in the body, which is contrary to the needs of our time.

We'd been working in the clinic for several years by then, and we already had around 80 patients coming every day. This was a good number, and gave us great experience, from which confirmed that the traditional formulas had many shortcomings. What we found is the following.

Firstly, the classical remedies are not so fit for modern times which are more Pitta-Vata. We live a life which is too aggressive, too fast, too full of stress and anxiety, which causes many illnesses connected with low Agni, low digestion, low immune systems. The classical formulas don't take care of these issues. In the time of more Kapha diseases these formulas were Pitta-Vata enhancing and not so suitable for our age and needs.

Secondly, classical formulas contain a lot of heavy metals, which I didn't agree with. I believe that we are organic and must take only organic natural substances, made from plants. So I decided to modify all the formulas to make them suitable for modern times, according to our experience working in the clinic.

Thirdly, most of the classical formulas are based on powders, so if you want to give the correct herbal dose to people, a combination of perhaps 10 herbs, two to three grams a day, then it becomes too much to handle. And if you give those same powders in the form of 300 mg tablets, then it's just one-tenth of a dose, which doesn't have any impact, it's not effective.

Being a pharmacist, I realised that we needed to extract the essence of the herbs, and if done in the right way we can then give the right dosage in just one 300 mg tablet, which is what is required to bring about the required transformation.

So this is what I did, following those principles. I started working on the formulas, creating new ones, and tried them out for two or three years to a group of people without charging them, observing the whole clinical impact on them and finalising what was effective.

Following this process, by 1992 I had created 80 different formulas, which were first based firstly on making sure that Pitta and Vata were not increased, and secondly that each and every formula, even if it is for skin disease or anything else, should improve health in general.

Nowadays people often don't move their bodies that much; we are immobile, sitting in offices all day. We are stressed, have no time for exercise, so our both our digestion and metabolism are very slow. Most people, when they are working, just run from one thing to another, and they grab whatever food is available on the run. This combination of the wrong food, no exercise and lots of stress completely depletes our digestive and metabolic enzymes; it dries out the enzyme secretion in the body, causing illness and poor health.

Thirdly, what we do has to have a real effect, using powerful extracts of herbs which really work to resolve the problem that we are addressing; if the problem is a cough, then it has to resolve that issue; if it is a skin problem, then it has to resolve that.

Fourthly, we must work to remove blockages in our systems; we are constantly blocked up by toxins in our bodies. We gradually pile up these toxins, little by little, drop by drop, over a period of years. We are often not aware of this until it emerges in the form of the sudden symptom of a major illness.

Often we wonder what we did wrong just yesterday to bring about this illness, what we did two months ago to merit a heart attack. But it's not like that. In truth our heart attack has been building up over the last ten years, not the last two or three months. What we need to do is to remove the blockages and toxins which have built up in the minute tissues within the channels within the body.

I followed these principles and created formulas that were truly effective. In fact we found them to be remarkably good, and the results were so striking that patients started referring people to us in large numbers. People started talking about us by word of mouth and our practice grew from 80 patients to three or four hundred a day in our Ayushakti clinics.

Ayushakti was formed as a company in 1988. By 1992 I had worked for six years on creating different herbal formulas. My work began to increase. Besides the formula work I was handling the whole of the business, I was handling the whole leadership of the organisation, alongside my own practice twice a week, and also had developed a complete Panchkarma detox model based on pulse readings.

Additional to the three focuses of pulse reading, Panchkarma and herbal formulas comes the fourth: diet. By following a specific diet for the improvement of the quality of your life, around half of all illnesses disappear.

These are the four areas that I focused on, and which became my areas of true expertise.

By 1998, Dr Pankaj and I had started travelling to Europe. The first country we came to was Italy. We met lots of doctors there, and gave lectures to them, sharing what we can do with them, and four of these doctors came to study with us in India. This is how we began working in the West.

Taking my time, working with the authorities, we started exporting herbal products to Europe in 1990, first to Italy and then to Germany and other places. From this beginning I have now travelled around the world doing pulse reading; in Europe, America, Australia and New Zealand and Russia—and of course, India.

I have seen so far, around 300,000 new clients on a one-on-one basis. Most of them suffer from chronic pain, arthritis, spondylosis, frozen shoulders, diabetes, high blood pressure, high cholesterol, severe obesity, IBS (irritable bowel syndrome), chronic digestive disorders, asthma, allergies, coughs and colds. I have helped a lot of people who have been suffering from cancer to prevent its recurrence for at least 15 years.

Other health issues include; ulcerative colitis, psoriasis, hair loss and baldness, alopecia, eczema, children's eczema, and other children's problems such as low concentration, hyperactivity, autism, limited growth in children, and many, many other health conditions where Ayurveda can help.

The key is pulse reading, which is a diagnostic technique that gives an understanding of what's happening behind the scenes, and how long this has been invisibly cooking away. For example, somebody has a sudden health problem, say a heart attack. Why did this happen? What had been going on behind the scenes over the years to cause it? And if you want to prevent it in the future, you have to deal with the cause of the problem in the past, or it will recur.

Pulse reading tells you exactly what went wrong in the hidden past, as well as what is happening now. It tells us what is happening right now in the body, the mind and the emotions, which indicates what should be prevented today to avoid problems in the future. Pulse reading is both an art and a science of observation and insight

I have seen, by training more than 60 doctors in pulse reading, that the more a doctor practices, the more insight they gain. Today, in every Ayushakti clinic in India, we have around 80 to 100 patients coming every day, which means that when people come to study they have lots of practical pulse reading, practical hands—on experience, and they become sharper, sharper, sharper with practice.

From all this experience I want to share with you the principles of Ayurveda in a down to earth, practical way. I will do this by telling you of the experiences people just like you and me have had, how their health was greatly improved, and how you too can make a difference to your own life and health

This book is divided into three sections:

1. **Ayurveda in Action.** This section demonstrates by the use of real people's stories how the principles of Ayurveda have made a great difference to their health. This section will give you an understanding of the essence of Ayurveda, including the special terms we use.

2. **Treating Common Ailments.** The core of the book. Here we look at eleven of the most common ailments we see in Ayushakti Clinics, with practical, proven solutions we have to make a real difference ourselves, as well as working directly with Ayushakti clinicians.

3. **Diet, Health and the Stages of Life.** Insights from my observations and experience into the profound effect our diet has on the state of our health, with reference to the changes we need to be conscious of in the different stages of our lives, from young to old.

# Ayurveda in Action

Reading what has actually happened to real people who have used Ayurveda to eliminate disease is the best way of gaining understanding and confidence in the power we all have to assist the process of returning to health. Before you read these stories, or start using the guidance in the main section, you need to understand some principles we use in Ayurveda that have no equivalent in English, so we use the traditional words. You will find them throughout this book because there is no other way to express some ideas precisely. Becoming familiar with these special terms also opens us to understanding our bodies and health in another way.

## The Three Doshas

Ayurveda believes that there are five elements which are at the essence of the entire universe, both animated, as in you and I, and non-animated, such as the planet we live on. These elements are; space, air; fire, water and earth, and within our bodies they combine to create what we call the three *doshas*, qualities or energies that influence all our bodily functions; *Vata, Pitta* and *Kapha.* Understanding the essence of the three doshas, and the other terms you see below is necessary for making sense of all that is written in this book.

## VATA

Vata is composed of space and air, and is the subtle energy in the body which is associated with movement and change. It governs, for example, breathing, the beating of the heart, all muscle movements and the fine actions that take place at the cellular level. When this dosha is in balance it leads to creativity and flexibility; when out of balance it leads to anxiety, fear, dysfunction, pain and stiffness.

## PITTA

Pitta is composed of fire and water, and is at the essence of the metabolic system, the workings of our bodies such as digestion, absorption, assimilation and the governing of body temperature. In balance, Pitta promotes understanding and intelligence, and out of balance it creates excessive anger, frustration and irritation, skin problems, acidity, and inflammatory disorders in the body.

## KAPHA

Kapha is mainly composed of earth and water, and as such is the energy which forms the structure of the body. Kapha is the source of lubrication for the body, and keeps the joints flexible and the skin moisturised, as well as maintaining our immune system. In balance, this dosha promotes love, forgiveness and stillness; out of balance it leads to greed, attachment and possessiveness. Too much Kapha causes excess mucous and, for example, heart diseases which are associated with congestion in the arteries.

## AGNI

Agni is the metabolic fire, the body energy that at a physical level is entirely responsible for transforming things from one form to another, in all the steps from food to tissue. Every transformation is supported by Agni, which is therefore vital for health, because every function of our body is founded on change—from food to cells, from air to energy and so on—and if Agni is diminished, then so are all our functions.

## AMA

Ama is the name Ayurveda gives to the toxins in the body which are associated with undigested food, ingested pollutants, or experiences that are not assimilated within our minds. Excess Ama leads to our bodily systems being clogged or blocked, because it is not excreted by our natural systems. It leads to fermentation and subsequent imbalance in all three doshas. Ama, toxic material, is fertile ground for the development of disease. It has no useful function within the body, only destructive, so is best avoided and removed.

## SROTAS

Srotas are physical channels within the body, from large such as the digestive tract, to the microscopic, at the cellular level. Srotas carry blood, sweat, pancreatic fluid, semen, faeces, and are the means by which nutrients reach our cells, and the means by which we excrete waste. To keep these channels open and flexible is naturally an essence of good health.

## DHATUS AND OJAS

Agni digests whatever we eat and coverts it into nutritional plasma and faeces. The lymph and the blood stream absorb the nutritional plasma and transform them into various tissues with the aid of Dhatu Agni (metabolic fire). Normally the transformation process occurs in the following sequence:

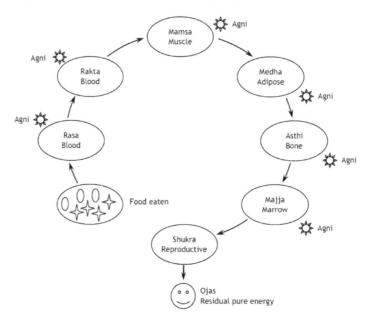

Food eaten nourishes the Rasa (plasma) and, with the aid of Agni, it is transformed into Rakta (blood). The process continues with Agni acting on the tissue at the stage of conversion.

Ojas is generated at the end of the conversion process, which is the residual pure energy vital for maintaining the immune power of the body.

Healthy Dhatus and Ojas promote positive emotions, immunity, vitality, strength, health, enthusiasm and tranquillity of mind.

# Stories of Ayurveda in Action

Now I will share with you four stories of patients of mine which tell you very much about the wonderful way that Ayurveda works to restore health. Each of these stories tells you about a different aspect of typical ailments that we encounter in our lives at this time, and how health was restored to these patients in ways I have seen to be effective, time after time. I've changed the names of the patients to respect their privacy, but their stories are unchanged, and real.

## JACK

*The experience of a man who suffered from depression, obesity, chronic fatigue, diabetes and high cholesterol, who restored his health through Ayurveda.*

Jack, who came to see me in California, tells a typical story of our time. He was 6'2 " tall and weighed 230 kilos, had problems with high cholesterol, diabetes, depression, and had retired prematurely because he was suffering from profound chronic fatigue. He could no longer work, and was being financially supported by his family.

When I checked his pulse, I found extreme levels of Ama toxins in his body, and his metabolism and digestion were depleted. Extremely high Vata was rising to his head, and this made him feel light-headed. To compensate, he ate lots of food to give himself a sense of grounding, and over time he grew bigger and bigger.

His is a typical story. When he was young he was slim and very fit, did lots of sports and was very active at school. And, of course, he loved food. As his parents didn't have time to cook, he ate pizzas and burgers and chips and all sorts of junk food every day of his life. But, at that time, he did at least one hour of sports every day, so he never gained too much weight.

Then, when he was around 24 years old, he graduated from university and started working for his family business. He now spent his life sitting at a desk, without physical exertion. He worked hard every day, from 8 in the morning until 8 in the evening. It was an import-export business where he spent his days on the phone or talking to clients, sometimes going to their warehouse by car. So he hardly moved his body at work, and had no time to exercise because he was so busy.

But he still ate the same food that he loved in his youth; pizzas and burgers and pasta and other refined foods, the things that can create Ama. But now he wasn't exercising, he was hardly moving, and on top of this he had lots of stress from his work which led to his digestion not functioning as well as it should. Stress impacts on digestion very badly, and of the three kinds of stress—mental, emotional and physical—emotional stress is by far the worst. Every year he put on five kilos, then another five, but he didn't pay it much attention as he was growing very gradually, bit by bit. Over ten years he went from 80 to 130 kilos.

Then, when he was around 34, he suddenly felt drained and weak. He collapsed, almost fainted, and he was taken to the hospital emergency room. The doctors did a complete check-up and found that he had very high blood sugar levels. The doctor told him he had to take powerful medication immediately, to bring his blood sugar level down, otherwise he would go into a coma. So this is what he did.

He was not aware at all of what was good for his health. Lack of exercise, along with eating heavy, poor food, produced half-digested toxic Ama and these toxins were blocking channels within his body, and producing a lot of gas after eating. All of this was going on behind his diagnosed diabetes, and he kept on eating the same junk food.

It's easy for people to live like this; junk food is available, tasty, and heavy, so you feel grounded and a bit better, for a while. But if you don't exercise and live with high stress you can't properly digest that food, and it produces toxic Ama.

That Ama blocks many, many channels within our bodies. If it goes into the pancreatic system, for example, it produces Type 2 diabetes. The pancreas produces insulin but it's not released because there is a blockage in a channel. Or the toxin goes into your arteries in your head or leg or main artery, where it can produce a thrombosis, a heart attack or atherosclerosis.

If it gets into the mental channels, then this Ama causes confusion, lack of mental clarity and lethargy. People feel very tired all the time and don't want to do anything, there is no clarity about what to do, despite a lot of mental activity.

If this Ama stays in the digestive tract, whatever you eat is not absorbed because it blocks the absorption of nutrients, and the result of low absorption is chronic fatigue. Whatever you eat, no matter how nutritious, doesn't get into your blood system because it's not digested and not absorbed.

According to Ayurveda, Vata, the vital air, is totally responsible for creating essential movement in our bodies, but when this Vata rises up into the head because of blockages, it causes light-headedness, depression, and stress. Jack, at the age of 36, weighed 230 kilos, with Type 2 diabetes and high blood pressure. He was completely depressed and chronically tired because whatever he ate was not absorbed well. He felt he could hardly work at all because he was so exhausted, both mentally and physically. This meant he couldn't work anymore and became dependent on his family.

He tried lots of diets with the intention of losing weight. Each time he dieted he did lose weight, but always put the weight back on as soon as he stopped dieting. This was because nothing affected the depression, stress and anxiety which were the cause of Jack eating so much in the first place. Significantly, nothing really worked on stimulating metabolism and digestion at the root level, encouraging the enzymes that are required to process nutrients.

I talked to him about the whole concept of Ayurveda; about digestion and metabolism improvement at the root level so that you stop producing fat, and keep your ideal weight rather than putting weight back on again. He was fascinated, and started following a specific diet plan, alongside specific herbs to work on his anxiety, depression, stress, and food addiction, to remove the toxic mucus of Ama from his bodily channels, and to enhance his metabolic enzyme production.

In the first six months he lost around 18 kilos. He was quite impressed. Once in a while when he didn't follow the diet, he didn't put the weight back on again, so he gained a little faith, and he came to India for Panchkarma. Through this detoxification process, we removed all the toxic mucus, Ama, and we stimulated his enzymes and metabolic structure completely. In one Panchkarma, we gave him around 30 different enemas, and with each enema he lost one kilo; 30 kilos overall.

Then I guided him in how to take care of himself. We created a two and a half year plan, during which he essentially restored his original metabolism and digestion. Then he restored his mental state through diet, Panchkarma, herbs and kitchen remedies, and using marma points.

Following this regime he lost around 150 kilos over two years. Since then he has maintained his weight for almost 20 years, and got rid of his Type 2 diabetes. He learned how to manage himself, so he exercises every day, and constantly detoxes as part of his lifestyle process. He has learned that if he eats something wrong, he can follow it with a kind of fasting over the next two days to balance the ill effects. In this way he has managed to keep his weight stable at around 80 kilos, and has managed to handle other aspects of his health, such as depression. His sugar and cholesterol levels remain under control naturally. As his story is typical of many people in our time, many of us have much to learn from it, both in the causes of his ailments and the solution to them.

## RITA

*The experience of a woman who suffered from early onset osteoporosis, exhaustion, and early menopause, who regained normal bone density and energy levels through Ayurveda.*

Rita was born and brought up in California. At the age of 48 she had an extremely high Vata constitution; she was very thin, and her mind was constantly racing from one thing to another, never stopping, which led to her not sleeping well at night. She is a typical example of imbalanced Vata. Her appetite was irregular; sometimes she ate a lot and sometimes she didn't want to eat at all. When she did eat a lot she never gained any weight, and she looked very, very skinny, even bony. And she was exhausted all the time. She had a lot of initial energy but very soon, within an hour, she would feel exhausted and need to rest. Her menstruation stopped when she was just 42; which is too young. Slowly, little by little, the hormones were not there to support her, and in consequence her metabolism and Agni were not working properly.

Agni, as the digestive enzyme, is responsible for breaking down the food and converting it into liquid and then finally converting it into nutritional plasma. The next step is creating bodily tissues on a daily basis. Millions and millions of cells die and have to be reproduced. This happens with the help of different enzymes and hormones. According to Ayurveda, they are converted, step by step into seven levels of tissue; plasma, blood, and so on. Plasma, which is known as rasa, completely controls thyroid functioning, lactation, pituitary hormones and hormone secretions for female and male reproductive systems. So if rasa is not nourished properly, there will be imbalance in these essential hormones. The next level is rakta—blood tissue—which is responsible for several other functions in the body, each of which is possible only when there is proper Agni present and functioning in the body.

Rita had a problem that because her Vata was so high, her Agni was completely depleted. To understand this, imagine Agni to be like a fire, a kind of liquid fire in the body. Agni comes out of Pitta. Note that the doshas Pitta-Vata-Kapha are responsible for our basic anatomy and the physiology of the body. They are the energies behind everything that happens in our bodily system, they are vital energies. All three are necessary for our bodies; we need them. But if any one of them is in excess, it causes problems.

Imagine Agni as being a kind of liquid hot Pitta energy converted into enzymes and hormones, which are always working away as catalysts for millions of different processes within our bodies. This means Agni is like a fire, and if you think of softly blowing on a candle flame, it burns more strongly with the added oxygen, but if you blow it too hard the flame goes out.

In the case of Rita, the excessive air element, Vata, in her system, had blown her Agni out almost completely. Because she had too much air in her body she had practically no Agni. She was born with a high Vata constitution, and on top of that there was an additional Vata imbalance because of her age and contributing hormonal factors.

Stress was the other contributing factor to her high Vata. She had had such a traumatic experience of marriage, which ended when she was around 30 or 32, that she never formed any further close relationships. She became dried up because she was alone, all by herself, with no companionship.

In time, after turning her attention to the spiritual, she became very strong as one of the leaders of a very big spiritual movement. This gave her some fulfilment, but then she became overactive because she wanted to remain busy. Only then she could she forget her inner loneliness.

She became overactive, working too much, endlessly travelling in the name of spreading her spiritual path. She didn't do this for money; she was a woman on a mission. This led to her creating even more Vata because she travelled by air every two days from city to city for her work, and air travel creates Vata, by its nature.

Her work gave her satisfaction, but her lifestyle was creating even more Vata, adding to the Vata in her constitution. This, along with the fact that her hormones had dried up by the age of 42, created trouble in her bones.

She was taking calcium as medication for osteoporosis but her bone density never improved; it stayed really low, and of course she wondered why. The calcium was not being converted into bones because her Agni was not working, and if the Agni is not working, nothing works. Even if you eat the richest nutrients in the world they aren't converted into tissues, and finally the tissues diminish. So if Agni is not working properly, the brain tissue diminishes, and this leads to Alzheimer's, or another type of memory loss. Another example of this, particularly in women, is that assimilation of calcium does not take place in the bones, so no matter how much calcium you eat, drink, or take in infusions. The result is osteopenia, osteoporosis and finally osteoarthritis.

My treatment for Rita was as follows. I gave her lots of our Ayushakti herbs to stimulate her Agni, along with castor oil to drink at every night with half a glass of warm water for months on end, which calmed down her Vata. I also told her to drink ghee, one teaspoonful of ghee on an empty stomach in the morning with ginger tea or fennel tea, and that also helped calm down her Vata.

If you put oil in a fire, it burns brighter. If you blow air into a fire in a controlled manner, it also burns brighter. Rita had the strong air of Vata blowing on and depleting her Agni for all 47 years of her life. We added oil to that process, and slowly, slowly—because obviously you can't create a miracle in one day—she felt the change coming step by step. We also gave her herbs to increase her Agni, and oil for nourishing that Agni, which reduced and calmed the Vata.

Finally, after some months, she became really convinced of the validity of Ayurveda, so she came to India for a full four weeks Panchkarma programme, where we also gave her lots of Bastis—enemas, oil enemas. We gave her lots of oil to drink too. She had ghee and oil coming into her from every doorway into her body; she was soaked in oil. The oil came from massage, from drinks, from enemas—from every direction. After four weeks of oils and different herbs to increase her Agni she felt like a completely different person. She felt very grounded, less nervous, very energetic, more stable in her thinking, and slept well for the first time in 20 years.

I also gave her lots of natural seashell and other organic forms of calcium that her body could absorb easily. After three months of this she had a bone density scan, and for the first time ever her density rose.

It is possible if you follow the right process, to reverse what is happening behind the scenes in a body, step by step, and this is what happened to Rita. In time she reduced her high Vata and restored the effect on her Agni; she digested her food well and became calmer, more balanced and happier.

## LUIGI

*The experience of a man whose life was limited by chronic acidity, migraine and anger, and found a new lifestyle through Ayurveda.*

We have a doctor in Italy, Dr Sebastiano Lisciani, who has been practising Ayurveda successfully since 1990 with Ayushakti, and has lots of patients. He comes from Sicily which is, as you know, in the South of Italy. It has a reputation for gangsters and the mafia, and one mafia boss who had a specific issue with high acidity and headaches came to see Dr Lisciani, checked his pulse and found he had extreme high Pitta, which caused the acidity, the burning sensations, along with occasional skin eruptions.

Italians love eating tomatoes of course, which increase Pitta greatly. So this man Luigi had high Pitta, acidity, constant headaches, two or three times per week. Dr Lisciani advised him to reduce his Pitta enhancing diet, the sour food, tomatoes and so on, to diminish his high acidity and headaches. He also gave him herbs to reduce the Pitta in the head region, bring it down and remove it through his daily bowel elimination.

After four months this patient came back to Dr Lisciani and said, 'I want my money back! 'Dr Lisciani was very surprised and asked him, 'What happened, don't you feel better? ''It's not that, 'said the patient. 'I no longer have headaches and high acidity, but I still want my money back.'

Dr Lisciani asked, 'If you got the result you wanted, why are you so unhappy? 'The patient replied, 'You know what, I get no headaches, have no high acidity, but my problem is that I'm not getting angry any more. I'm in a profession where I have to shout at people a lot, get angry with them to show my power, and I can't do that anymore because I'm not getting angry inside myself. So this treatment isn't helping my profession.'

Dr Lisciani said, 'Yes, your Pitta has diminished, so your anger is also diminished, along with your headaches and acidity. Now you have a choice. If you want your anger, you will also have headaches and acidity because even by getting angry you encourage high levels of Pitta.'

The man considered this for a while, and then said, 'The truth is that I'm in a much better state of being when I don't get angry all the time. My body feels so much better too, so I think, in time, I'll choose a new profession, one I don't have to get so angry in.'

That is the story of a man who reduced his Pitta to get rid of headaches and acidity, but also moved into changing his lifestyle by moving past his need to be angry. It clearly shows that our personality and our lifestyles have such a strong effect on our health and state of being—and that Ayurvedic treatment is powerful enough to bring about change at the deepest level of the way we live our lives.

## Mr Sharma

*The experience of man who suffered from obesity, and took control of his life and tendency to gain weight through Ayurveda.*

This is the story of Mr Sharma from London, which tells us something specific about Kapha. He weighed 140 kilos and was only 5'3 'tall, so he looked a bit like a little elephant. The reason why this is significant is that people nowadays who know something of Ayurveda often think that when someone tends towards being overweight they are more Kapha, but it's not necessarily true.

A real Kapha person is always happy and stable, would not quit but be committed to their partners, their relationships, their jobs; they stick to whatever they decide to do. They don't give up on things easily. That's a typical Kapha character.

I would say 80 per cent of the time these days people become obese because they have a high level of Vata in their bodies. This begins with a sense of insecurity, sadness and depression, quitting one job for another, not feeling happy at all in life, being dissatisfied with their partner but not trying to work things out with them, just imagining that they will change and all will be well.

People like this become very insecure in themselves, and because of that insecurity they have a craving to eat too much, often a craving for sweet foods, because they only feel very stable and grounded when they eat sugar. After many years of eating these things, they grow very large. This is a typical low metabolism and high Vata type of obesity.

In women, most of the time, a hormone imbalance can bring about an extreme level of water retention, which also creates a bloated feeling and looks like obesity, of a kind that doesn't diminish even with exercising or diet. It goes down only when you reduce Vata. This kind of person is not Kapha dominant. This is what I want to make clear, because many times when people who have this kind of weight issue read books about Ayurveda and think, 'Ah, I am Kapha, 'and then start eating all kinds of raw food and other specific foods, which works to increase Vata, These people become more nervous because of this then they eat more and, of course, they don't actually lose any weight.

Coming back to Mr Sharma, he was the most typical Kapha person I have ever seen in my life, one of the 20 per cent of obese people on this planet who have real Kapha obesity. This man was always happy; in every situation he found himself in he kept smiling all the time. He had a very clear vision for his business and was very successful. Temporary defeats never stopped him from doing what he wanted to do. He was also extremely flexible and had lots of energy. People who have a Vata kind of obesity have extreme low energy, they feel tired two to three hours after starting anything, whereas this man, even though he was obese, was so energetic he could dance so lightly that you couldn't believe he carried so much weight.

He was a typical Kapha kind of a person; very flexible, light and extremely energetic; he could work 14 hours a day, and at the same time gained weight very easily. Just by eating a little extra he could gain two kilos in two days. It was very difficult for him to lose weight because, typically for people like him, he loved eating, particularly crunchy fried Indian foods, not sweets in his case. For this reason it was difficult for him to lose weight.

In order to control his obesity he needed to activate his metabolism, at least two times his present rate, and process all that extra Ama toxins and fats so could become slim and get rid of his tendency to gain weight. We started periodical detox of five weeks, once a year, followed by seven days detox every two months. This removed his toxins and activated his metabolism very quickly. In that first year he lost thirty kilos. Also in that year, we gave him herbs and a specific diet to reduce both Kapha and Ama and activate his metabolism. In one and a half years he came to a point where he didn't gain weight easily and he knew if he ate something wrong how to balance it immediately.

This is a good example of a typical Kapha person. This demonstrates the point that Kapha, Pitta and Vata dominant people behave in a very specific ways. A Vata person's desk is always disorganised, with a lot of paper strewn all over the place. They are highly creative, full of vision and imagination, but they have no clarity when it comes to the execution of their visions. They can be great artists, but their energy can drain away very quickly.

A typical Pitta person is very organised, very structured in the way they speak, they are very good at making things happen. A Kapha person may also be visionary, but also brings stability to the whole team. If somebody has lost the point of a meeting, he'll bring him back in line. He can also hold Pitta and Kapha energy. Typically, he's a leader who can work with different mindsets and has enormous energy, he can work for 12 or 14 hours straight. When there is an argument, when there's disagreement in a meeting, the typical Vata person will say, 'You're wrong, but I doubt my opinion is right. 'A Pitta person will say, 'I am right and you are wrong. 'A Kapha will say, 'You are probably right and maybe I am right too, let's examine what is actually correct for this situation.'

## Mr Patel

*The experience of a man who overcame his high blood pressure and removed the blockages in his arteries.*

I want to share you the remarkable story of Mr Patel, from Mumbai, who had a heart problem. He really believes in Ayurveda, and has been following it for more than 27 years. He has been coming to Ayushakti, to me and my husband, to take care of his health through Ayurveda.

He became a very successful politician and began to work very hard and travel a lot; too much in fact, and in his business forgot about following a good diet. He ate whatever he could get on the road, all kinds of junk food, fried food, samosas, pakoras, and wheat, which I told him not to eat after 50, but he did anyway. He suffered from high blood pressure, which he controlled exclusively with treatments and herbs and diet from Ayushakti. He always controlled his naturally; he didn't need any medication from the doctor. For a few months, he could not exert himself, he felt breathless and had some pain in his chest. But one day he felt a severe chest pain on his left side, radiating from his shoulder to his hands. He felt pressure, squeezing, choking, numbness, with severe palpitations. Finally he fell unconscious and was taken to an emergency clinic. The doctor performed angiography, and three blockages were found.

The doctor told him, 'We must put a stent in that main artery—you will have to have surgery, if not today then soon. 'Mr Patel said, 'I don't want surgery, I'll just go to Dr Naram and do whatever she says. So he came straight to Ayushakti and we put him on a very strict diet, what we call Ama-reducing, blockage-reducing. This was a very, very strict detox diet, which I have seen completely restore heart function.

First, two days of fasting on ginger water, sliced fresh ginger in hot water, then just cooked vegetables because they have a kind of fibre which dissolves easily in blood and in turn dissolves the plaque in blood vessels. It is very difficult for most people to follow this diet, but this man was persistent. I told him to stay on vegetables exclusively for three months; breakfast, lunch and dinner, without carbohydrates such as potatoes, rice, wheat, bread, chapattis, or pasta. I also told him to eat a little mung bean soup just once a day.

Following this I said he should mostly eat vegetables, vegetables and more vegetables, specifically leafy green vegetables, a little carrot and more zucchini, pumpkin, and the Indian vegetable called loki, lots of squashes, and leafy greens. I told him he could eat them in any form, he could make them into a cutlet to eat in the morning, he could sauté them, they could come as they are, and if he got hungry he could eat vegetables, no fruit, no carbohydrates, seven times a day if he wanted. Because he was using to drinking chai I said he could have chai or coffee just twice a day, with less milk or no milk at all. He followed this regime seriously for two to three months along with heart dhara, which is a treatment on the heart to clear blockages. You make a circular well on the chest around your heart region out of dough, and then you pour a specific herbal concoction and oils into it. This helps to clear the mucus and blockages from that area. We also gave him a Basti, which is a kind of enema specifically designed to remove blockages. If you have this enema twice a week it removes the mucus—like blockages from your body little by little, through a process of elimination.

At the beginning of the treatment he could hardly manage 10 steps without feeling breathless. After three months of this treatment he could walk two kilometres without a problem. At this point we felt in his pulse that he was really much better, so he could now go and get another check-up. So he had a test, which was confirmed with an angiography, and to the doctor's surprise his 60 per cent arterial blockage had been completely dissolved, and the one on the side artery which had been 80 per cent blocked had diminished by 40 per cent. He then continued eating only protein and vegetables for the next three months—no carbohydrates—to dissolve the remaining 40 per cent.

This is a good example of the way the blockages, caused by Ama, create a lot of trouble in the body, and when you dissolve them you can slowly restore your health and improve your quality of life.

These real-life stories show a range of typical health problems in our day and age, and how Ayurveda worked to create real and lasting solutions to them. In each of these cases the self—effort of the patients made a large contribution to the restoration of their health. In the next section, the core of this book, I will show you what you can do to make a real difference to your health and your life by applying the principles that make a profound difference to all of us.

# Treating Common Ailments

## Introduction

This section is divided into twelve of the most common ailments that we encounter in our Ayushakti clinics at this time. I am sure that many of the health problems that concern any of you will be covered in principle here. Each of the 11 chapters gives detailed advice following the Ayurvedic practice which we have seen time after time make a real difference to the health of those people who follow the guidance that is offered.

For Ayushakti supplements and clinics, see page iv.

Notes for measures in ingredients:

g = gram

tsp = teaspoon (approx 5 ml)

tblsp = tablespoon (approx 15 ml)

green gram is the alternative name for mung

These ailments are as follows:                    (page)

Each of these subjects starts with a short introduction, demonstrating the practical effectiveness of both the efforts people have taken to enhance their health, backed by professional Ayurveda care from myself or other practitioners. These introductions to the effectiveness of Ayurveda are followed by the heart of this book, this is how you can take your health in your own hands. I am going to share with you how to take care of your health and how to improve your quality of life using the six tools of Ayurveda which are:

- Diet
- Lifestyle
- Home remedies
- Ayushakti herbal remedies
- Marma
- Panchkarma

# 1.  Joint, Back and Neck Pain

## Arthritis, Osteoporosis, Spondylitis, Sciatica, Nerve Pain, Back Pain

Mrs D, who lived in Canada, had suffered with severe rheumatoid arthritis for more than ten years, taking all sorts of painkillers, and had been given the maximum dose of steroids to suppress her immune system, and this was impacting on her liver. It was so bad that she could hardly walk. She was tired all the time, and just wanted to live a normal life, without using high dosage medication.

She called me when I was in Los Angeles and when I told her that I would need to check her pulse, she said she couldn't travel to meet me because her feet were so swollen and her joints so stiff that she could barely move around the house.

It was evident to me that she had a high level of Ama, toxic swelling, so I said that the best thing to do was to fast, to start with ginger water—a glass of hot water with a teaspoon of fresh ginger root ginger—and drink this every time she was hungry, this would burn the toxins and give her energy. Also she could apply a warm mix of ginger and flour and water to any place on her body where there was swelling, to let it dry and then remove with warm water. She did this two to three times a day.

In addition, she took castor oil, a tablespoon in hot water, because it removes Ama and Vata toxins from the stool. Excess Vata goes into the spaces in the joints and causes stiffness and pain, discomfort, low flexibility, and wherever Ama accumulates in the body it causes a very thick, mucus filled, inflammation. Through fasting alone, all these things can be greatly alleviated. For the next three to four days I told her to eat only mung and vegetable soups, as well as continuing with ginger water.

Through following this regime, in only three or four days, the swelling diminished by around fifty per cent. In ten days she was flexible enough to fly to see me in Los Angeles. I checked her pulse and she had severe rheumatoid arthritis.

I gave her a strict regimen of eating only mung and vegetable soup for five days a month: no wheat, nothing fried, no red meat, no yogurt or other fermented foods. All of these kinds of food cause inflammation in the body. On top of that no salad, no beans, because they are gas-creating foods, and too much gas also causes stiffness in the joints.

Generally at Ayushakti we can treat such problems with herbal remedies such as Painmukti, Sandhiyog and Sandhical together with diet, but in her case her illness was so chronic and deep that I told her to come to India for Panchkarma. The lady who couldn't move out of her house found the energy and capacity to fly to India, by following my instructions.

We gave her a very severe Panchkarma with Virechan and Basti, to remove all the toxins in the body, moving them into the digestive tract, and then with specific enemas and purgation processes removing them completely.

When these toxins had been expelled from her system we gave her specific process for building up her bony structures, and she became stronger and stronger. Because of the Panchkarma the toxins had been removed and her metabolism was now stronger, so that nutrients were now being well absorbed, and calcium was absorbed into her bones.

Two to three years later she no longer needed herbs, and her ten years of suffering were over.

## Guidance for the Relief of Joint Pain: Including Sciatica, Stiffness and Swelling, Nerve Pain, Neck and Back Pain

### DIET

Joint pain, swelling and stiffness are the direct result of the increased movement of Vata (air) in the body. A moderated diet which decreases Vata can help to relieve these conditions.

**Avoid foods which increase Vata**

Wheat and all wheat products, yoghurt/curd (dahi), tamarind (imli) and tomatoes, oily food, raw salad, red meat and fermented food like idli, dosa, gas-forming pulses like kidney beans (rajma), chickpeas, dry peas, white bean.

Chilled water, aerated drinks, cold milk, ice cream and all cold food and drink. Vata is cold and warming foods/drinks counterbalance.

All of these foods, if eaten regularly, lead to an increase in Vata which can decrease digestive power, ultimately producing toxins.

**Avoid red meat**—occasionally eat chicken and turkey, eggs and sometimes seafood.

**Avoid brassicas unless** using asafoetida or fenugreek as they are too gas forming.

## Eat more foods which pacify or reduce Vata

Grains and pulses: brown and white rice, Amaranth and rye, millet, mung beans, red and yellow lentils.

Vegetables: most vegetables, favour root vegetables, and green leafy vegetables. Always eat cooked vegetables.

Spices and herbs which stimulate Agni and are warming without aggravating Pitta like: ginger powder, garlic, clove, cinnamon, black pepper, cumin, cardamom.

Fruits: all sweet fruits including avocado, apricot, sweet grapes, sweet apple, pears, fresh figs and dates, berries.

Other foods: use honey, jaggery (palm sugar or slow-grown sweet syrups like molasses, date syrup, agave. Ghee—use freely as it carries qualities of other foods deep into tissues and detoxifies, butter and organic milk.

Soaked nuts—favour almonds and brazil nuts. Avoid peanuts, and eat other nut butters a couple of times a week.

**Calcium (Ca).** You should also ensure a daily intake of at least 1200 mg of calcium rich foods such as the following.

| Food | Ca content (mg per 100 g) | Preparation |
|---|---|---|
| Amaranth grain | 47 | |
| Dried curry leaves | 830 | make paste or chutney and use in the food |
| Sesame seeds | 100 | use 100 g paste from sesame and in the soup or like a spread |
| Cumin seed powder | 100 | mixed with jiggery can be used for high calcium intake from cumin |
| Poppy seeds | 100 | 100 g soaked seeds made into paste, can be used to make gravy of vegetables instead of using crème |
| Milk | 100 | |
| Spinach | | 1 cup boiled spinach has 245 mg of calcium |

## RECIPES TO IMPROVE DAILY CALCIUM INTAKE

### 1. Sesame Balls: Total calcium 150 mg each ball

| | |
|---|---|
| Sesame seeds | 50 g |
| Dates (seedless and chopped) | x 2 |
| Almonds | 15 g |
| Jaggery | 35 g |
| Cardamom powder 1 pinch | |

Roast and crush sesame seeds and almonds. Grate or cut jaggery into small pieces, add a little water and cook to softball stage. Add crushed sesame and almonds, then add chopped dates and cardamom powder. Mix well and remove from heat. Take teaspoonful and roll into balls. Store in fridge and have 1–2 daily.

## 2. Sesame Coriander Chutney/Spread: Total calcium—202 mg

| Sesame seeds | 15 g |
|---|---|
| Cumin seed | 2 pinch |
| Dry kokum/mangosteen | x 2 |
| Pomegranate powder | 1 tsp |
| Green chilli (optional) | x 2 |
| Coriander leaves | 20 gm |
| Curry leaves | 1 sprig |
| Root ginger (grated) | ½ tsp |
| Mint leaves | 1 sprig |
| Rock salt as per taste | |

Roast sesame and cumin seeds. Chop ginger and chilli. Wash the curry, coriander and mint leaves. Put all ingredients into a blender and grind until it turns into a chutney. You can use it as a spread on crackers or chapattis.

## 3. Calcium rich sauce for vegetables: total calcium 300 mg

| Sesame seed | 10 g |
|---|---|
| Poppy seed | 10 g |
| Red pumpkin/butternut squash | 5 g |
| Onion | 10 g |
| Kokum/dried mangosteen | 5 g |
| Ginger/garlic paste | 1 tsp |
| Coriander powder | ¼ tsp |
| Cumin powder | ½ tsp |
| Red chilli powder (optional) | 1 tsp |
| Turmeric powder | 2 pinch |

| | |
|---|---|
| Garam masala | ¼ tsp |
| Whole mung flour | 10 g |
| Ghee | 15 g |
| Salt as per taste | |

Soak sesame and poppy seeds in water for half an hour. Blend and boil it until it reduces to make a runny paste. Heat the ghee in pan and sauté ginger/garlic paste. Add all other ingredients and the sesame poppy mixture and cook till it becomes a light brown colour. You can add mixed boiled vegetables of your choice. Use this gravy.

## LIFESTYLE

- 30–45 minutes of daily exercise such as walking and swimming makes a great difference.
- Practice Pranayama and Anulom-Vilom (alternate nostril breathing) with the help of a yoga teacher.

### Further recommendations:

- Avoid over-exertion
- Avoid frequent late nights
- Learn to diminish the effects of worry, grief and fear, perhaps through meditation.

## HOME REMEDIES

- Drinking one teaspoon of castor oil with warm ginger water before going to sleep is a very effective way of keeping joint pain and arthritis at bay.
- Juiced white radish leaves (daikon radish) in the morning, during winter months

**Home remedy for pain relief**

| | |
|---|---|
| Turmeric (haldi) powder | 1 tsp |
| Dry ginger (sunthi) powder | ¼ tsp |
| Ajwain powder (wild celery) | ¼ tsp |
| Asafoetida (hing) | 1 pinch |
| Fenugreek seed powder (methi) | ½ tsp |
| Coriander seed powder dhania | 1 tsp |
| Garlic juice | ½ tsp |

Mix all these with water and take twice a day. In cases of severe pain take it three times a day, or as often as necessary.

**Joint pain in old age**

This type of pain is not necessarily due to arthritis, but general wear and tear over time.

**1.**

Take 4 tsp of ground sesame seeds daily.

**2.**

100 g rajigro—amaranth grain, per day.

**3.**

| | |
|---|---|
| Dry ginger powder (sunthi) | ¼ cup |
| Fenugreek seed powder (methi) | 2 tblsp |
| Ghee | 2 tblsp |
| Jaggery | ⅓ cup |

Mix the ingredients well and make the mix into half inch diameter balls. Store them in the fridge. Eat one ball each daily in the morning. This helps with back pain.

## AYUSHAKTI HERBAL REMEDIES

Proven and effective herbal remedies from Ayushakti to relieve joint pain, swelling, arthritis, sciatica, spondylitis, osteoporosis.

### Painmukti MJ tablets

To relieve back pain, neck pain, joint pain, frozen shoulder, sciatica, muscular pain, for stiffness pain and swelling.

**Dosage:** For minor and recent pain one tablet 3 times a day. For chronic and severe pain: 2 tablets twice a day for 3 to 6 months.

### Painmukti Sandhi-Cal tablets

Calcium supplement for your bones, for Vata reduction.

These tablets effectively reduce bone degeneration, and cracking of the joints. Relieves osteoarthritis and osteoporosis.

### Dosage:
- For stiffness and cracking in joints: 1 tablet twice daily to prevent bone degeneration and relieve stiffness and pain.
- For chronic pain and stiffness, osteoporosis and back pain: 2 tabs twice daily.
- For those aged over 60: 2 tablets twice daily to keep your joints nourished and free from pain and stiffness.

### Painmukti Cream

This cream contains Mahanarayan Oil combined with powerful pain-relieving herbs and other oils, proven to provide faster and 3 times longer-lasting relief than any other cream.

Application: Apply 4 times a day. For minor pain continue for a week. For chronic pain, continue for two months. After this, apply it whenever necessary.

## MARMA

### Pindswed

Of the various kinds of Panchkarma therapy for different health concerns, pindswed improves flexibility of joints, relieves arthritis, swelling, sciatica and spondylosis.

### Instructions for pindswed

Mix one cup of ajwain powder and one cup of dry ginger powder. Divide into two equal parts and tie in thick cotton cloths to make two pouches of equal size. Heat one ball on a dry skillet or iron. Apply this heated ball to the painful areas for at least twenty minutes and apply Painmukti Cream thereafter.

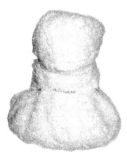

**A pindswed ball**

## ARTHROX

Arthrox is a powerful detoxification programme which can relieve the root cause of any chronic ailment. A full Arthrox first removes toxins from all bodily channels through purgation therapies and herbal enemas. This is followed by Rasayana, a rejuvenation program which helps nourish the tissues and cells and prevents degeneration. After a full Arthrox, you will feel lighter, more focused, with joints free of pain, and walk and stand without pain.

*For Ayushakti supplements and clinics, see page iv.*

# 2. Skin Disorders and Skin Care

## Acne, Psoriasis, Eczema, Urticaria/Hives

One of the daughters of a family who regularly came to the Ayushakti clinic was getting married in three weeks, and she was going out shopping in Mumbai every day in preparation. Now the food is great in Mumbai, and when you go out shopping like that, you eat out, of course. That food tends to be full of tomatoes, and much of it is fermented and fried and oily; all high in Pitta.

Suddenly, after a week of this her face broke out in acne. Here she is getting married and her face was full of acne. This created a lot of stress, because in India the bride has to look beautiful, but she was looking terrible.

So she came to see me and her pulse showed very high Pitta. She told me she'd been eating a lot of tomatoes, lemons and vinegar, fried and fermented foods in the last seven days, lots of it.

She started immediately eating mung and vegetables only, because with this diet toxins begin to move out very quickly, Ayushakti Virechan tablets to remove all the toxins from her body, and specific face pack treatments described later in this section.

I gave her a smart detox programme over seven days. You do lots of fasting with mung and vegetable soup, and at night take herbs which expel mucousy, hot toxins from the body completely, along with high dosage purgations, and in four or five days her Pitta diminished and her acne subsided dramatically. She was surprised and very pleased. Her face became clear, and she was the most beautiful of brides on her wedding day.

### Sam from New Zealand

When I met Sam in 2010 almost 70 per cent of his body was covered with psoriasis and he was constantly scratching his itching skin. He was using cortisone cream to keep the itching at bay, and had been suffering with condition for more than twenty years; it was almost intolerable.

Now psoriasis is a condition which arises from extremely high Pitta and an hyperactive immune system; it's an autoimmune disease. When the immune system is overactive it attacks the skin, which becomes inflamed, which leads to dermatitis, psoriasis and other skin conditions.

When I took his pulse I found a hyperactive immune system, with lots of heat, high levels of Pitta. I told him that it would take a very long time, you can't expect any magic solution here, but over time, month by month, year by year, you will find it improving so you will be able to manage without cortisone cream.

For the first three years he took herbs and home remedies; one teaspoon of turmeric twice a day, and his diet should be Pitta reducing—nothing sour, no vinegar, tomatoes, lemon and no wheat or milk, which can also trigger the inflammation process, and no red meat.

He followed this regime religiously, taking three to four herbal skin tonic tablets twice a day, 2 D-Vyro tablets twice a day for immune balance.

He did this for three years, religiously, and quite a lot disappeared. He had fewer attacks and hardly needed steroid creams at all. Finally I said he should come to India and do Panchkarma for four weeks. During that Panchkarma he expelled lots of yellow mucus during the day of purgation, and every day felt lots of hot toxins moving out of his system.

Following that I gave him a skin rejuvenation and immune-building programme for him to follow at home, with high dosage of herbs, following the Panchkarma process. After two months of this his skin became fabulous, soft and supple as a child, he hardly needed any creams at all. To this day he maintains this skin, taking some herbs and following a clear diet.

## Guidance for the Relief of Skin Disorders

Reducing and eliminating the Pitta (heat) in the body is very important in the treatment of skin disorders. Generally, people who have chronic skin disorders should follow a strict diet. Those with minor skin disorders should avoid sour foods like tomatoes, lemons, vinegar, tamarind, citrus fruits, and fermented foods. The sourness in amla, pomegranate, kokum, and mangosteen are exceptions to this rule.

### DIET

The skin mirrors the inner condition of the body.

When the Agni (digestive fire) is weak, food does not get digested properly. The undigested food then causes Ama (toxic mucous) and excess doshas, especially Pitta (heat). The excess heat gets absorbed by the blood and circulates throughout the body and gets gradually deposited in the blood tissue and muscle tissue. When toxins are not eliminated through the digestive system, they can be thrown out through the skin, resulting in rashes, boils, pus, itching, dark patches, or skin infections and diseases like eczema, psoriasis, dermatitis, etc. Reducing and eliminating the Pitta (heat) in the body is very important in the treatment of skin disorders. Generally, people who have chronic skin disorders should follow a strict diet. Those with minor skin disorders should avoid sour foods like tomatoes, lemons, vinegar, tamarind, citrus fruits, and fermented foods. The sources in amla, pomegranate, mangos teen, and kokum are exceptions to this rule.

### Avoid foods which aggravate Pitta

Fermented food like pickles, idli, and dosa; desserts involving fermented processes.

Pungent vegetables like brinjal, chillies, capsicum, tomatoes, fenugreek leaves, asafoetida; cucumber, radishes, okra, raw carrots.

Sour fruits like lemons, oranges, grapefruit, pineapples, sour cherries, sour plums, sour grapes, peaches, mangoes, strawberries.

Alcohol, vinegar, colas, hot chocolate.

Yogurt, buttermilk, cheese, eggs.

Millet, refined white flour, wheat, cashews, peanuts, kidney beans, chick peas, dried peas, black eyed beans, tamarind, white broad beans,

Seafood, fish, lobster, red meat, beef, veal, pork.

Particularly avoid mixing foods that are not compatible, such as milk with meat, milk with fish, milk with fruit, milk with honey, or milk with salted food or sour foods.

### Eat more foods which pacify or reduce Pitta

Sweet fruits like coconuts, figs, apples, sweet black grapes, melons, sweet oranges, pears, pomegranates, resins, sweet and bitter-tasting vegetables like cauliflower,

French beans, peas, potatoes, all the squashes and pumpkins; barley, rice, corn, white meat, egg whites, etc.

Rice, barley, oats, mung, mung dal, lentils, red lentils, pumpkins, squashes, fresh peas, cooked onion, sweet potato, fresh corn, leafy vegetables, lettuce, all sweet fruits, grapes, bananas, watermelons, sweet melons, figs, coconuts, avocado, sweet apples, honeydew melons, fresh olives, pears, warm milk with cardamom, fresh cheese like cottage cheese, ginger, fennel, cumin, coriander, cinnamon, almonds, sweet fruit juices, those desserts made with rice, milk, cream and sugar. Generally, it is recommended to eat more soft vegetables with a high water content, such as squashes, white and red pumpkin, spinach, etc. Use ghee liberally in place of oil.

## LIFESTYLE

- Avoid over-exposure to sun and wind, smoking and late nights.
- Only eat when hungry, don't eat when you're not hungry. Refrain from eating when stressed, anxious or angry.
- Don't wear synthetic clothes or use chemical cosmetics,
- When you wash your face, allow the water to dry naturally so that it moisturizes the skin.

### Exercise

Exercise improves circulation, helps remove toxins from the body, stimulates growth hormone levels and decreases destructive stress-hormone levels. In this way, exercise goes a long way toward helping slow down the aging process

## HOME REMEDIES FOR SKIN DISORDERS

### 1. For reducing Pitta, and calming skin problems

| | |
|---|---|
| Raisins soaked overnight | 20 |
| Cumin seed powder (jeera) | ½ tsp |
| Coriander seed powder (dhaniya) | ½ tsp |
| Fennel seed powder (saunf) | 1 tsp |
| Turmeric powder (haldi) | 1 tsp |

Squeeze the juice out of the soaked raisins or, simply add the other ingredients and blend. Drink it twice a day.

### 2. For eliminating excess heat and toxins

| | |
|---|---|
| Haritaki (Terminalia chebula) | 100 g |
| Castor oil | 10 g |
| Ajwain seed powder (owa) | 20 g |
| Black salt (sanchal or kala namak) | 10 g |

Mix all ingredients together and keep bottled. Take one tsp with water daily, every night before going to bed.

### 3. One tsp of ghee with warm milk on an empty stomach early every morning.

Ghee calms down the Pitta in the body.

### 4. One tsp of turmeric powder (haldi) twice a day with water.

Helps reduce skin allergies and infections.

### 5. Body rashes due to Pitta

Apply kokum oil (garcinia) or fresh kokum water or ghee on the rashes.

### 6. Urticaria, itching and hives

| | |
|---|---|
| Ghee | 1 tsp |
| Black pepper powder | ¼ tsp |
| Ajwain (owa) seed powder | ¼ tsp |
| Jaggery (unrefined raw sugar) | 1 tsp |

Mix them together and take in the morning on an empty stomach. If needed, take twice daily.

*or:* Apply ghee all over the body, especially on the rashes. For better results use Ayushakti Sudarun body lotion.

### 7. Psoriasis

| | |
|---|---|
| Ghee | 100 g |
| Turmeric powder (haldi) | 10 g |
| Liquorice powder (yastimadhu) | 5 g |
| Sesame oil (tila taila) | 30 ml |

Warm the ingredients and massage the affected areas with it. Repeat 2–3 times per day.

### 8. Eczema

| | |
|---|---|
| Fresh or dried neem leaves | 10 |
| Water | 1 glass |
| Turmeric powder | 1 tsp |
| Triphala powder | 1 tsp |

Mix well and take at night.

**9. Dry eczema**

| | |
|---|---|
| Neem oil | 1 tsp |
| Karanj oil | 1 tsp |
| Pure ghee | 1 tsp |
| Sesame oil | 1 tsp |

Mix well and apply 3–4 times per day.

## Acne

When boys and girls reach 12–14 years of age, hormonal changes often result in acne on the face. Sometimes, it goes away in a year or two. But often it can stay until the 30s. In some women, acne may return when menopause begins. Acne occurs as a result of too much heat in the body. From my experience I have seen that acne can be completely relieved if Pitta toxins are diminished.

**Treatment for Acne** involves reducing Pitta and Ama. Along with this, one should also avoid external heat.

**Diet and lifestyle to eliminate acne** should include following a Pitta and Ama-reducing diet to balance the doshas, pacify the Pitta and reduce Ama.

**Important:** Do not squeeze pimples, because this can spread the infection, causing more pimples and possibly scars.

**Face pack treatment for acne**

Mix together:

| | |
|---|---|
| Coriander seed powder | ½ tsp |
| Sandalwood powder | 1 tsp |
| Vacha (calamus root) powder | ½ tsp |

| Nutmeg powder | ¼ tsp |
| Multani mitti (fuller's earth) powder | 1 tblsp |
| Sandalwood oil | 3 drops |
| Rose water | 1 tsp |
| Enough water to make a paste | |

Apply the face pack after taking a facial steam bath every day or every other day. To take a steam bath bring water to the boil, take it off the heat, then cover your head with a towel, lean over the water and allow the steam onto your face for a while. When your face is dry, wash it with cold water.

## AYUSHAKTI HERBAL REMEDIES

**Ayushakti Skin Tonic.** Two tablets twice a day for 6–12 months clears the skin from acne, pimples, skin allergies, infections, dermatitis. For chronic diseases like psoriasis, eczema, warts etc, need to take the tablets in double dose for 2 years or more as per the skin conditions

**Ayushakti Rupam Cream.** Apply cream on acne and scars at night, leave it overnight and wash it off in the morning.

**Ayushakti Sudarun Lotion.** Contains Mahatikta Ghrut (medicated ghee) and herbs. It calms heat when applied on skin very effective for psoriasis, eczema, dandruff, hives.

## SKINOTOX

Detoxification is very important in all types of skin disease. Virechan and Basti in Skinotox effectively reduce the excess heat and toxins from the body and help the skin to return to normal slowly and steadily.

Detoxification treatments are done in Ayushakti clinics worldwide.

# Skin Care

As we grow older, Vata increases, depleting the skin's moisture and oil. Excess Vata also blocks regeneration of the skin. Thus the process of shedding dead skin and generating new skin slows down. Consequently, the skin begins to look rough, lifeless and wrinkled. However, with the wisdom of Ayurveda, it is possible to prevent and delay this aging.

## DIET

The skin always reflects the internal condition of the body. By following certain dietary instructions along with external applications, you can purify your skin from within and look youthful and radiant.

Reduce the amount of heavy beans such as kidney beans, chickpeas, dried peas, etc.

Reduce gas-causing vegetables such as cabbage, cauliflower and salads.

Reduce heavy meats such as pork and beef.

Eat more soft vegetables with a high water content, such as squash and pumpkins, spinach and leafy greens.

Drink lots of fruit juice and eat fruits during the day.

Use ghee liberally with your meals instead of oil. Ghee is traditionally known for its anti-aging properties.

## LIFESTYLE

- Avoid excess exposure to the sun and wind.
- When you wash your face, allow the water to dry naturally so that it can moisturize the skin.

### HOME REMEDIES AND HOMEMADE SKINCARE TREATMENTS

One teaspoon of ghee on an empty stomach with warm water or milk early in the morning.

One teaspoon of turmeric powder twice a day with water.

### 1. Homemade cleansing milk

| | |
|---|---|
| Marigold petals | 2 tblsp |
| Charoli seeds (Buchanania lanza) | 1 tsp |
| Ritha (soapnut) | 1 whole |
| Honey | 1 tsp |

Mix with enough water to make a thick liquid

Soak charoli seeds and ritha in water for four hours. Blend all the ingredients with a little water. Filter and squeeze the juice. Add enough water to make a thick liquid. Smear it all over the face and wipe with wet cotton. Keep it refrigerated.

You can use this cleansing milk every evening to remove makeup, dirt and pollutants from the face.

## 2. Natural toner for glowing skin

| | |
|---|---|
| Milk | 1 tblsp |
| Almond milk | 1 tsp |
| Ghee | ¼ tsp |
| Corn starch | 1 pinch |
| Sandalwood oil | 5 drops |

Soak two or three almonds in water. Peel off the skin, add a little water and crush them in the blender. Filter and squeeze the thick almond milk. Heat the ingredients, except for the sandalwood oil, till the cornstarch dissolves. Cool it and add the sandalwood oil. Apply to your face before going to bed. Leave it overnight and wash it off in the morning. Alternatively, apply it in the morning and wash it off half an hour later.

## 3. Body scrub

| | |
|---|---|
| Chana dal (bengal gram) coarsely powdered | 1 cup |
| Masoor dal (red lentil) coarsely powdered | ½ cup |
| Turmeric powder | 2 tblsp |
| Sandalwood powder | ¼ cup |
| Coriander seed powder (dhaniya) | ¼ cup |
| Red sandalwood powder | ¼ cup |
| Milk cream | ¼ tsp |
| Enough milk to make a paste | |

Mix the dry powders together and keep this mixture bottled. Mix a handful with a quarter teaspoon of milk cream and enough milk to make a paste. Scrub your body and face regularly by gently applying this mixture onto the skin. It will remove dead cells, stimulate blood circulation and generate a youthfully radiant skin.

### 4. Nourishing face cream

| | |
|---|---|
| Banana pulp | 2 tblsp |
| Ghee | ¼ tsp |
| Sesame seed powder | 1 tsp |
| Almond milk | ½ tsp |
| Aloe vera juice | ½ tsp |
| Water and milk | |

Soak one almond in water for two hours. Remove the skin, add one tablespoon of water and blend it in the mixer till it becomes a fine liquid. Filter. Blend the other ingredients in a blender by adding enough milk to make a smooth paste with a creamy consistency. Keep it refrigerated. Massage gently into the skin.

### 5. Face pack

| | |
|---|---|
| Multani mitti (fuller's earth) powder | 2 tblsp |
| Coriander seed powder (dhaniya) | ½ tsp |
| Sandalwood powder | ½ tsp |
| Liquorice powder | 1 tsp |
| Honey | 1 tsp |

Mix well with milk to make a paste. Apply mixture all over the face and allow to dry.

### 6. Home facials—the Ayurvedic way

Every week, after the age of 40, follow this simple home facial process. Between the ages of 30 and 40, do it once every fifteen days.

### Step 1

Use the homemade cleanser from the Homemade Cosmetics section. Apply the cleanser and remove it with a wet cotton swab.

**Step 2**

Apply the Ayushakti Glowing Body Scrub or the body scrub from the Homemade Cosmetics section all over the face and neck. Let it dry. Massage gently with wet hands and wash your face with water. This process will remove dead skin and stimulate the generation of new skin.

**Step 3**

Massage your face and neck for 15 to 20 minutes with Ayushakti Nourishing Night Cream or the Nourishing Cream Formula given in the Homemade Cosmetics section. When you massage your face, begin by rubbing ice all over your face to nourish and refine your skin. Gradually, fine lines and wrinkles will begin to disappear. The massaging action will also promote blood circulation under the skin.

The massage will take around 15 to 20 minutes. Watch yourself in the mirror as you follow the instructions.

Apply the cream sparingly all over your face.

On your forehead, gently apply the cream upward from the eyebrows toward the top of the forehead for about two to three minutes. You should feel your skin being pulled upward. With your index finger, form the figure eight all over your forehead for a minute or two.

Pinch your eyebrows with your index finger and thumb, moving from the centre to the edges. Do this for a minute or two.

Use your index, middle and ring fingers to massage your eyeballs, moving from the centre upward and outward in a circular direction and covering both eyes completely. Do it for two to three minutes. Pat your eyes very gently with your fingers two to three times. Cover your eyes with your four fingers and hold it for a few seconds. Do this two times.

By using your index and middle fingers, massage your nose on both sides from top to bottom. Move your fingers downward in a circular motion for two to three minutes.

**Cheeks**

Using your index fingers, massage from the bottom of your nose toward your ears in a circular motion for two to three minutes.

Using all four fingers, massage your cheeks, beginning at the centre and continuing in a circular upward motion over the entire cheek. Do this for two to three minutes.

With your three middle fingers, massage from the base of your nose toward your ears. Gently pull your skin outward and upward for two to three minutes.

Pat your face all over with your fingers for two to three minutes.

**Chin and jaws**

Hold your chin with your index finger and thumb on both sides. Pinch your jaws from one end to the other for two to three minutes.

**Lips**

With your index fingers, beginning at the centre of the upper lip, gently massage outward around the lips for a minute.

Hold your lips with your index and middle fingers. Pull your lips from end to end for a minute.

Smile Lines—Keep your index fingers flat on your smile lines. Move them upward and downward for a minute.

**Neck**

With the four fingers of both hands, massage your neck from bottom to top in an outward motion, gently pulling your skin for two to three minutes. Stop massaging when you feel the cream has been absorbed.

**Step 4**

Inhale steam with your head wrapped in a towel. The steam can be taken by using home sauna equipment or by using water boiling in a vessel. The steam opens the pores so that toxins under the skin are released and blood circulation improves.

**Step 5**

Apply Ayushakti Rejuvenating Face Pack or a face pack from the homemade cosmetics section and let it dry for 15 to 20 minutes. When it dries completely, wash it off with cold water. Do not wipe your face with a towel. Allow the water to dry naturally so that the skin absorbs moisture from the water. The pack nourishes the skin, tightens the pores and restores the normal texture of the skin, particularly in older people.

Following this regimen regularly prevents aging, by gradually refining the skin, removing wrinkles and fine lines, and restoring youthful skin.

## Removing Skin Pigmentation

After the age of 40, the skin may develops pigmentation as a result of hormonal changes and excess Vata and Pitta which in turn lead to degeneration of the skin. Very often, toxins block blood circulation beneath the skin, causing dark patches on the cheeks or forehead.

## HOME REMEDIES

**1.**

| | |
|---|---|
| Turmeric powder (haldi) | 1 tsp |
| Red sandalwood powder (chandana) | ½ tsp |

Drink with half glass of water twice a day.

**2.**

| | |
|---|---|
| Red sandalwood powder (chandana) | 1 tsp |
| Turmeric powder (haldi) | ¼ tsp |
| Ghee | ¼ tsp |
| Multani mitti (fuller's earth clay) | 2 tblsp |
| Honey | ½ tsp |

Mix them well and apply the mixture like a face pack. Let it dry and wash. Do not wipe with a towel; rather, allow the skin to absorb the water. Do this three to four times a week.

## AYUSHAKTI HERBAL REMEDIES

- Apply Ayushakti Protective Day Cream two to three times a day.
- Apply Ayushakti Nourishing Night Cream every night before going to bed.
- Take Ayushakti Skin Tonic Tablets.

# Clearing Blackheads with Ayurveda

Excess Pitta and Ama generate toxins which accumulate in the pores of the skin. These toxins dehydrate and ooze out when you press the pores. Very often, the skin pores explode. Dirt and pollutants from the air are deposited there, causing blackheads. After a steam black grains pop out, if you press them. If you do not cleanse them, you see many black dots on the face.

## Treatment

Internal treatments include purifying the skin and reducing Pitta and Ama is necessary to remove blackheads. Externally, the pores of the skin need to be cleansed.

### HOME REMEDIES

Take one teaspoon of turmeric powder (haldi) twice a day with water.

Steam your face very well. Using a small cotton pad, press the blackheads with your index fingers in order to remove the black grains. Then apply the following pack.

| | |
|---|---|
| Masoor powder (red lentil) (coarsely powdered) | ¼ cup |
| Sandalwood (chandan) powder | 1 tsp |
| mango seeds without the hard skin (Ama guthali) | 1 tsp |
| Turmeric powder (haldi) | ¼ tsp |
| Rubia cordifolia (manjishta) powder | ½ tsp |
| Jasad bhasma | ¼ tsp |
| Liquorice powder (yastimadhu) | ½ tsp |
| Pipal leaves juice (Ficus religiosa) | enough to make a paste |

Mix the ingredients well and make into a paste. Apply the mixture to your face and allow it to dry. Rub it off with wet hands and wash. Lightly massage your skin with the ice cubes. Wipe with a towel.

**Note**: Manjishta, jasad bhasma and jeshtimadhu can be found in any Ayurvedic store.

## Astringents

Astringents are required to tighten the pores. Aging and excess Ama dilate the pores.

In order to prevent blackheads, pores need to be tightened.

| | |
|---|---|
| Cucumber juice | 1 tblsp |
| Marigold juice | ½ tblsp |
| Rose water | 1 tblsp |
| Katha (very fine powder) | ¼ tsp |

Mix the ingredients. Refrigerate and use it for two to three days. With a cotton swab, apply it on the face after cleansing. Allow it to dry for 10 to fifteen minutes. Wash it off with water. You can also apply it after taking a bath or washing your face in the morning.

### AYUSHAKTI HERBAL REMEDIES

**Ayushakti Mukhkalp** face pack prevents blackheads.

Use **Ayushakti Skin Tonic** tablet for healthy skin.

**Ayushakti Gentle Face Wash** acts as an astringent.

# Daily Routines for Smooth, Youthful and Glowing Skin

To keep your skin youthful, you need to follow certain simple daily and weekly routines. The daily routines are all the more applicable for dry, aging and lifeless-looking skin.

- Apply Ayushakti Protective Day Cream two to three times a day to protect the skin from the sun, dirt, pollution and wind. If applied daily, it nourishes the skin and removes wrinkles.
- Cleanse your face with Ayushakti Gentle Face Wash instead of soap to moisturize your skin naturally.
- Cleanse your face twice a day with the homemade cleanser described in the Homemade Cosmetics section.
- Massage your face and neck every night for 10 to fifteen minutes with Ayushakti Nourishing Night Cream or Nourishing Cream given in the Homemade Cosmetics section.
- Two to three times a week, apply Ayushakti Glowing Body Scrub with milk on the face and body. Allow it to dry on the face for a while and wash it off with water. Smear it gently all over the body and take a bath. Alternatively, you can use the body scrub described in the Homemade Cosmetics Section.

*For Ayushakti supplements and clinics, see page iv.*

# 3. Stress and Depression

This story of John from New York is a good example of the effectiveness of Ayurveda in dealing not only with stress and depression, but a range of mental issues which had plagued him for a lifetime. He suffered for years from Attention Deficit Disorder, he had learning disabilities, his memory and focus were poor, and he was hyper-active.

Instead of enrolling in a special school, handling his mental issues with prescribed tranquilizers, he started taking specific Ayushakti herbs, and his life changed dramatically over a period of two to three years. He felt he had become a different person, being listed in the first five in his honours program, and was looking forward to a fruitful life. His enthusiasm for Ayurveda—following his own real and powerful experience—was so great that he brought more than fifty friends and family members to Ayushakti.

It's also good to note that the story of Jack the previous section (see page 13) also demonstrates the powerful effect of Ayurveda on stress and depression, which was, as is often the case, part of a complex of health issues.

## DIET

Your diet needs to be a mixture of foods that increase both Rasa Dhatu and Ojas, while at the same time reducing Vata (air) and Ama (toxic mucous).

**Foods to avoid:** Raw vegetables, salads, eggplant, raw onions, peas, capsicum, potatoes, tomatoes, white sugar, wheat, red meat, sweets, fried foods and fermented foods.

**Foods to consume more of:** Organic milk, buttermilk, oranges, berries, pomegranates, passion fruit, cherries, raw cane sugar, cumin, grapes, millet, cotton seed oil, soybean oil, ghee, garlic, cumin, butter, sweet fruits like bananas, coconuts, figs, dates, grapes, melons, papayas, cooked vegetables, beetroot, carrot, garlic, French beans, cooked onion, cooked ladies fingers, sweet potatoes, all kinds of squashes and pumpkins like ridge gourd, bottle gourd, snake gourd, red and white pumpkin, cooked rice and eggs, aloe vera, asparagus, green dandelion, cantaloupe, mung beans, red and yellow lentils.

All types of nuts are good in moderate quantities as are jaggery (unrefined sugar available in Indian grocery stores), honey, palm sugar, and ghee (also available in health food and Indian stores). All kinds of oils are permitted in moderate quantity. Vegetable juices, chicken, turkey and seafood are permitted in moderate quantities. To get vitamins from raw food, drink juices (for energy) rather than raw salads (to avoid formation of gas).

## LIFESTYLE

- Your Lifestyle creates positive thoughts, and self-confidence.
- Close your eyes and observe your breath for ten minutes in the morning.

- Also practice Pranayama with the help of a yoga teacher.
- Light physical exercise naturally increases the body's cellular activities and thus strengthens the immune system. Exercising regularly will also help prevent illness and disease, so you can think of it as relaxation therapy!
- Physical activities that can be performed without a break for at least 12 minutes such as cycling, or jogging are call aerobic exercise. This is the best type of activity for increasing general levels of fitness—particularly the performance of the heart, lungs and muscles.

## HOME REMEDIES

### Digestive tea to increase Agni and metabolism

| | |
|---|---|
| Cumin seed powder | 1 tsp |
| Fennel seed powder | ½ tsp |
| Rose petals | 20 |
| Coriander seed powder | 1 tsp |
| Raw cane sugar | 1 tsp |
| Water | 1 glass |

Boil the above mixture and keep it covered for 20 minutes. Filter and drink. This will release extra VATA and calm anger, anxiety etc. and stimulate digestion.

### For all fear, depression and feelings of insecurity

½ cup juice of white pumpkin or Indian lauki

1 tsp Ghee in the morning on an empty stomach with warm water or herbal tea.

1 tsp Brahmi (Gotucola) powder (available in health and Indian stores) twice a day. Brahmi has the power to gradually reduce the production of stress chemicals in the

body—especially Cortisol—and increases and reinstates your body's natural immunity.

Soak 20 raisins in water for 3 hours, then crush and drink the juice. This will calm flared up emotions.

**For emotional upset following shock**

Sniff 1 grain of black pepper and 1 pinch of liquorice powder mixed together in both the nostrils once a day, to restore alertness and clarity.

Take 1 tsp ghee with warm milk or warm almond milk.

Take 1 tsp gotu cola powder twice daily.

**Powerful herbs which help release stress and strengthen your immune system**

These herbs calm down your emotions, increase immunity and allow your body and mind to respond calmly in any situation.

**Jatamansi** (Nardostachys jatamansi). Relieves deep-rooted tensions and helps to remove mental toxins and physical and mental strain.

**Ashwagandha** (Withania somnifera). This herb directly opposes the reactions of stress and anxiety by reducing the amount of Cortisol released by the adrenal glands. It encourages restful sleep, again helping the body to recover from the effects of stress, anxiety and depression. Ashwagandha lowers the blood pressure and it is highly effective in stopping the formation of stress-induced ulcers. Ashwagandha increases the number of immune cells known as T cells and B cells—helping to fight infections. All these actions directly oppose the harmful effects of stress. It is a strong anti-oxidant.

**Bacopa monniera.** Calms the heart, regulates blood pressure and is a nervine tonic that helps to release emotional blocks like stress, phobia, frustration and panic attacks. It is a strong anti-oxidant, creates focus and awareness.

**Ginger** (Zingiber officinalis). Increases metabolism, focus and awareness and gives mental equilibrium.

**Yashtimadhu** (liquorice). A strong antioxidant, calming, soothing and nourishes the tissues. It also improves focus and awareness.

## AYUSHAKTI HERBAL REMEDIES

**Bliss tablets and Suhruday tablets** improve circulation and metabolism, which in turn improves brain function and cell renewal. This helps to restore emotional balance, focus, awareness and mental well-being, increases alertness, concentration and memory. They also reduce fears, phobias, confusion, and negative thoughts by promoting Satvic qualities of mind. It is also anti-aging and antioxidant, and helps protect from memory loss due to aging. Bliss helps to create joy and happiness, reduces fear, insecurity, and gives confidence.

## MARMA

Marma techniques are very effective if done in a specific manner and with great focus. These subtle energy points can create a powerful impact in your mental channels to bring back positivity, concentration, self-confidence, happiness and zeal. Marma techniques help to remove blocks, reduce symptoms instantly, and nourish tissues.

### Massaging the soles of your feet

Foot massage with ghee is extremely effective in bringing Vata down from the head. When you massage ghee into the soles of your feet, your head immediately feels cool, focused and clear. This also stimulates circulation throughout the body.

### To release stress, anxiety, and depression: marma point for depression, anxiety, fear, panic attack and pain

Press marma point 7 located on the right arm. To locate this point, count six fingers up from the lines on the inner wrist as shown in figure 1, pressing with the index finger as shown in figure 2.

Benefits of this marma: This assists a person in feeling comfortable, happy, mentally and emotionally stable.

Press this point six times, six times a day, and when needed, as well.

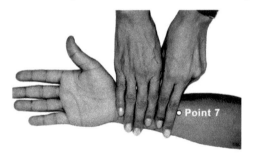

Fig. 1

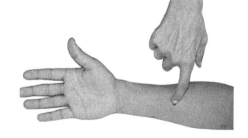

Fig. 2

## PANCHKARMA

Panchkarma is a purification process and one of the traditional limbs of Ayurveda treatment. This 5-week residential Ayurveda treatment programme completely cleanses and then rejuvenates the body, freeing the mind and emotions of toxins. Every individual patient receives a unique treatment combination of the five processes—according to their specific health needs.

Heart Dhara and Shirodhara are two of the treatments used in Panchkarma which are especially beneficial for reduction of stress, depression, phobias, fear, feeling of insecurity, irritation, mental pressure, and low self-esteem.

**Heart Dhara** is one treatment that expressly reduces fear, stress, grief and depression. Heart Dhara stimulates positive emotions like happiness, contentment, confidence, and security.

**Shirodhara** creates tranquillity. When a mental channel is nourished properly, you will remain calm, tranquil, and stable even in the most adverse situations. Shirodhara (see illustration below) miraculously creates tranquillity by eliminating agitation, nervousness, headache, insomnia and fear.

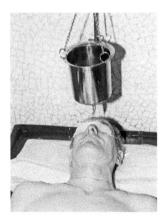

**Nasya** is the nasal administration of herbal oils and ghee. This treatment opens mental channels, and restores focus, concentration and awareness. With long-term use, it can also enhance memory.

**Note: Panchkarma treatments should be done with the help of a trained Vaidhya only.**

*For Ayushakti supplements and clinics, see page iv.*

# 4. Sleep Disorders

## Introduction

Sleeping well is one of the most important sources of good health, according to Ayurveda and common sense. We say there are three Stambhas, or pillars, that support good health; right diet, right sleep and right sexual discipline, so good sleep is vital to our lives. It reduces the effects of aging, improves fertility, memory, builds stamina, alertness of mind and prevents arthritis. Good sleep is to be valued highly. It is, indeed, a foundation of good health and happiness.

The best, healthiest sleep is 8 hours in a dark, silent room, ideally from around 10pm to around 6 or 7am. Many people in today's world go to bed late and wake up late. This means their deep sleep is much reduced. In addition to the length of time in bed, the quality of our sleep is vital. This means we often find problems with incomplete or poor quality sleep. The consequences are fatigue and clumsiness, along with feeling fatigued during the day, reduced performance, irritability, high blood pressure, weight gain and more.

To compensate by sleeping in the day is not advisable. The exceptions a young children and people over 60, for whom it is beneficial.

As a general rule, according to what we practise in Ayushakti, deep and sound sleep comes when Kapha is increased in the head region, which can be produced by drinking milk or ghee.

Typical causes of poor sleep and their solutions are as follows.

## Insomnia

One of the main causes of insomnia is anxiety, constantly worrying, which doesn't turn off at night; in fact it can increase. Other causes are joint pain, prostate conditions or urinary incontinence, for example. When we deal with those conditions, the insomnia is also dealt with.

A common solution to insomnia is to take sleeping pills. This kind of medication can not only become addictive, but also cause serious side-effects, so it should be avoided if possible.

I can give you an example from one of my own patients, which demonstrates the interrelation between poor sleep and other health conditions. This woman had suffered from poor sleep since she was young, and when she began an early menopause found things became worse. This led to irritability, depression, anxiety, and tension headaches.

Following the way we handle these issues in Ayushakti, the solution was found in relaxation in meditation, an adjustment of her diet, herbal remedies and home remedies. Within six months her sleep pattern changed entirely, and for the first time for many years she slept for seven to eight hours a night. This led to a profound sense of healing. Her experience of living was transformed.

If you have trouble sleeping, you must strictly keep to the following regimen:

- Go to bed and get up at a regular time, and very gradually make it half an hour earlier if you are used to waking late.
- Completely darken your bedroom with blackout curtains, and turn off the lights after 10 pm.
- Leave a gap of 45 minutes after watching TV before going to bed.
- Don't nap during the day unless it's absolutely necessary. Even then, restrict your nap to 15 to 20 minutes in the early afternoon.
- Get plenty of exercise during the day, but don't exercise in the 2 hours before your bedtime.
- Eat early in the evening. Avoid caffeine, especially after 7 pm. Try to avoid all beverages after dinner if you find yourself getting up in the night to urinate.
- Use this simple technique to prevent worrying at night: 1 hour before bedtime review and write down your problems in a diary. Think them over for 10 minutes, asking yourself; what I can do to resolve this? Write down all the solutions that come up. Close the diary and leave it to read it in the morning. This will help you to calm your mind down, let go of your worries, and help bring sound sleep.

## RECOMMENDED DIET TO ENCOURAGE GOOD SLEEP

mung; gourds (dudhi), parval, turai, tindali, spinach, methi, coriander, white and red pumpkin, French beans, carrots, beetroot, onion, garlic, ginger, zuchini (courgette), leafy green and cooked vegetables.

Ghee, kichadi, oats, mixed grain chapattis.

Avoid red meat, refined maida and deep fried foods.

## HOME REMEDY

| | |
|---|---|
| Pippali root powder | ¼ tsp |
| Milk | ½ cup |
| Sugar | ½ tsp |
| Ghee | 1 tsp |
| Nutmeg | 1 pinch |
| Tagar (valerian root) powder | ½ tsp |

Mix the ingredients with boiling water, let cool and drink it warm before going to bed.

## MARMA

For chronic insomnia; practicing regular shirodhara and using deep detoxifying enemas from Ayushakti will lead to profound positive results within 2 or 3 months.

Apply cow ghee with a kasa vati (small, shallow bronze bowl) to the soles of the feet at bedtime.

# Snoring

When someone snores it means they aren't sleeping deeply or well, making it a kind of sleep disorder. Nevertheless, many people who snore—who are usually men— think they sleep well despite their snoring. This is not true. The truth is that snoring comes from the lack of elasticity in a soft palate at the root of the tongue. This prevents food from entering the windpipe, which blocks the breath and causes snoring. This means that the problem with snoring is not just the noise, but the fact that the airflow is reduced to some degree. This leads to a reduction in oxygen intake, which in turn leads to waking up feeling sleepy and tired for the rest of the day.

At Ayushakti we deal with this with special home remedy—which you can see below. This will usually stop this problem within six months. A lifetime of snoring—with its effects on wives and others—can be stopped forever. The effect is powerful and liberating for everyone.

## DIET

Do not eat fried foods, milk products or red meat in the evening. These foods produce mucus which blocks the airflow and leads to snoring.

Take 1 teaspoon of ghee with warm water before going to bed. This reduces vayu, strengthening and toning the soft palate (uvula).

Following this simple method leads to a minimum reduction of 80% in snoring in three to six months.

# Sleep Apnoea

Chronic snoring can lead to the serious problem of sleep apnoea; blockages in the nasal airway leading to periods of interrupted breathing. The soft palate mentioned above, which closes the airway when we swallow, can close that airway during sleep. This leads to as much as 8 to 10 seconds without in-breath, which can give a sense of being choked, then waking up. This can happen as many as 30 to 40 times a night and a poor night's sleep. You can wake up feeling drowsy and irritable. Many years of sleep apnoea can lead to high blood pressure and strokes.

The common medical solution is by the use of machines. Many patients find them inconvenient, with limited long term effectiveness. They do not, for example, affect the sleep apnoea impact upon memory and performance in the workplace.

We deal with this issue at Ayushakti with a course of controlled diet, home remedies and herbs. We find this combination effective in restoring good sound sleep to those suffering from sleep apnoea within two or three months.

## HOW TO STOP SLEEP APNOEA

The most important thing is to get your weight under control. Cut down on carbohydrates such as bread, pasta, rice and wheat chapattis. Eat more vegetables and protein such as lentils, mung, legumes, eggs, tofu, fish or chicken.

Do not eat fried foods, wheat, milk products or red meat, as these foods produce the mucus which leads to snoring, and consequently sleep apnoea.

Recommended foods include jowari or ragi chapattis. Keep to a mung and vegetable diet for five days at least once a year, which will cleanse your toxins and remove blockages to breathing.

Take one teaspoonful of ghee with warm water before going to bed.

## HOME REMEDY TO EASE THE BREATH

| | |
|---|---|
| Bharangi | 1 tsp |
| Kantkari | 1 tsp |
| Piprimool | 1 tsp |

Mix the powders together and take twice a day for one year. This will help greatly with sleep apnoea.

Note: Sleep apnoea is a chronic problem; if you are using a machine to facilitate breathing keep on using it. At the same time follow the recommended diet and home remedies. Your sleep patterns will definitely improve within a few months.

# Restless Leg Syndrome

Restless Leg Syndrome (RLS)—moving our legs restlessly during sleep—is a disorder which originates in the nervous system. As it interferes with good sleep it is considered a sleep disorder. It most commonly affects the legs but can also affect the arms, torso, head and even phantom limbs.

Sensations related to RLS range from muscle pain to itching feelings, unpleasant tickles or even a 'crawling 'feeling. These symptoms typically begin or intensify during times of quiet wakefulness, such as when relaxing, reading, studying or trying to sleep.

It affects both sexes, but is more common in women.

### Why do we get Restless Legs Syndrome?

- Genetic; we inherit it from our family.
- Iron deficiency, particularly in women.
- Diabetes; as a result of diabetes.
- Medication; some types of medication, including some anti-depressants and some anti-histamines may worsen symptoms.
- Pregnancy; some women experience RLS during pregnancy, particularly in the last trimester. Symptoms usually go away within a month of giving birth.
- Other factors: alcohol use and sleep deprivation may trigger symptoms or make them worse.

### How to get relief from Restless Legs Syndrome

- Regular exercise, especially swimming, walking and yoga.
- Swimming and walking should be for 45 minutes three times a week.
- Yoga and Pilates based stretching exercises three times a week for 45 minutes each time.
- Reduce weight—eat mung soup and vegetables only for five days a month.
- Eat more protein and vegetables.
- Massage the legs with dry ginger and ajwain powder for 10 minutes before going to bed.
- Treat diabetes and arthritis naturally.
- Eat rice, yellow mung dhal, cooked vegetables, fruit and juices.
- Soak your legs in warm salt water before going to sleep.
- Practice backward bending yoga asanas to relax the nerves.
- Follow the recommended sleep regime (see above) to improve sleep.
- Eliminate alcohol.

### AN EFFECTIVE HOME REMEDY FOR EVERYDAY USE

| | |
|---|---|
| Piparimool powder | 1 tsp |
| Ginger powder | ¼ tsp |

Boil the above in half a glass of water and add 1 tsp of castor oil. Cool, and drink half an hour before going to bed.

### DIET TO REDUCE AMA

Your food intake should be in the following proportions:

| | |
|---|---|
| Vegetables | 50% |
| Proteins | 30% |
| Carbohydrates | 20% |

## Recommended diet

**Include:** mung beans, gourds (dudhi), parval, tindali, spinach, methi, coriander, white and red pumpkin, French beans, carrots, beetroot, onions, garlic, and ginger.

**Avoid:** wheat, meat, sweets, fried foods, fermented foods and heavy beans.

All the above are proven ways to eliminate Restless Leg Syndrome, which can cause real suffering without knowing how to deal with it. Following these recommendations really helps to get peaceful and sound sleep.

*For Ayushakti supplements and clinics, see page iv.*

# 5. Weight Reduction

## Weight Reduction

Obesity is the main epidemic in the world today. It is the leading cause of chronic illnesses such as heart attacks, diabetes, high blood pressure, urinary tract stones, arthritis, infertility and more. It is very difficult to effectively lose weight, and when we try and nothing works, we tend to stop trying.

Obesity is broadly due to having a very slow metabolism, having hormonal imbalance, water retention, or being bloated with air.

The cause and solution to obesity is distinct in men and women, and needs to be handled separately.

## Weight Reduction for Women

Many women gain weight quickly during transitional times in their lives, such as menarche—when periods begin—having a baby, or menopause. PCOS (polycystic ovarian syndrome) and thyroid imbalance may also have an effect on body weight. Despite doing lots of exercise and following strict diets, it can seem that nothing will actually reduce fat from the waist, tummy, thighs, chest and other places.

My experience in Ayushakti has given me proven methods of controlling your weight naturally. I am going to share with these with you in this section. If you follow the advice below—systematically and religiously—I am sure you will lose one to two kilos a month. You will lose inches from the difficult-to-change areas of your body. This will lead to you reducing 10 to 20 kilos in six to eight months. Additionally, you will find a bonus in the reduction of high blood sugar levels, a reduction in blood pressure, balanced hormone levels, and an easing of inner blockages, leading to an increase in fertility. Your skin will become softer, more supple, with fewer wrinkles, leading to radiance in your appearance.

**A SIX MONTH WEIGHT LOSS PLAN**

Begin with a 10 day detox program, as follows:

1.  For the first one or two days, take in only warm ginger water, one cup every half hour, and nothing else at all. To make ginger water mix ¼ of a teaspoonful of dry ginger powder in five glasses of water, bring to the boil and let it cool. This assists in melting fat, improving metabolism, leading to a sense of lightness and improved energy.

2.  For the next three days live on a mung and vegetable soup diet. To make the soup soak 1 cup (250 ml) of whole green mung overnight. Drain, add fresh water, salt and the spices of your choice. Cook in a pressure cooker with two cups (500 ml) of chopped vegetables—preferably leafy greens, squashes and pumpkins. Eat this soup warm, as many times a day as you want. You may drink tea once or twice a day rather than the soup.

3.  For the following five days, add more vegetable to the mung, to make it thicker, along with mung patties or pancakes. Recommended vegetables include

pumpkins, zucchinis (courgettes), kale, squashes, asparagus, leafy greens, broccoli, lauki, turai, tendli, and the padwal types of Indian vegetables.

4.    After 10 days of this regime, measure yourself and see the difference!

5.    From the 11th day onward, return to a normal diet, with the exclusion of fried, fermented and sour foods, wheat, red meat, cheese and yoghurt. Make sure that your diet is 60% vegetables, 35% protein (such as mung, lentils, tofu, fish, chicken, eggs), with a small quantity, up to 5% of carbohydrates such as rice, millet or potatoes. It's fine to completely avoid carbohydrates. Follow this diet for next 6 months.

If you follow this detox diet for 10 days every month, or even every two months followed by diet as per point no. 5 on all other days, without doubt you will easily gain control over your weight, and look younger at the same time.

## LIFESTYLE

It is critically important to have a regular exercise routine. Spend one hour a day exercising your body in the following way: 20 minutes of yoga or Pilates; 30 minutes of cardiovascular exercise such as running, cycling, swimming, dancing, or aerobics; 10 minutes of weight training.

## PRANAYAMA

**Anulom vilom:** 10 minutes every day

**Kapalbhati:** 10 minutes every day

Focus on yoga postures for thighs, tummy, butts, and tyre reduction. Consult a yoga trainer for yoga postures like:

**Utkatasan** (chair pose): 5 times a day

**Hastapadasan** (standing forward bend): 5 times a day

**Suryanamaskar** (sun salutation): 5 times everyday including all 12 yoga postures.

Also do **Bhujangasan** (cobra pose), **Naukasan** (boat pose), and **Salabhasan** (locust pose) each 5 times a day.

## HOME REMEDY FOR WOMEN WHO WANT TO LOSE WEIGHT

This home remedy really is amazing. If you take this regularly it will really help to remove swelling, melt fat and balance hormones. It will normalise your monthly cycle along with losing weight.

**To make barley water**

1 tablespoon full barley
3 Garcinia fruit (kokam)
2 (500 ml) cups of water

Cook this in a pressure cooker and filter.

Pour half of the mixture in one bowl and half in another. To one bowl of barley water, to drink in the morning, add and mix:

| | |
|---|---|
| Cumin powder | 1 tsp |
| Fennel powder | 1 tsp |
| Ajwain powder | ½ tsp |
| Asafoetida | 1 pinch |
| Dry ginger powder | ¼ tsp |
| Gokshur (Tribulus terrestris) powder | ½ tsp |

Make the mixture once more in the evening, using the remaining barley water, and drink it.

If you take this remedy every day you will easily lose two to three kilos a month. Many women I have known have lost up to 20 kilos in six to eight months. You won't believe how much more energetic you will feel, and how your face will glow. Of course, remember to follow diet of protein and vegetables only, and no more than 5% carbohydrates.

### AYUSHAKTI HERBAL REMEDIES

**Suhruday**: 2 tablets, twice a day—helps to improve the hormone and metabolic system. It also reduces mood swings, sadness, and stress.

**Ktone**: 2 tablets, twice a day—reduces water retention and feeling bloated. Flushes toxins through the kidneys.

**Mednil**: 3 tablets, twice a day—reduces fat and weight and makes you look slim.

## Weight Reduction for Men

Excess weight among men is always due to a sluggish metabolism, and only rarely due to thyroid or hormonal imbalance. Ayurveda believes that if the metabolic cycle is slow then even low calorie food can create excess fat. Additionally, when there is too much Vata—air—with high emotional and mental stress, too much thinking, sadness and fear leads to a tendency to eat constantly and thus put on weight easily. A sedentary lifestyle, stress, and eating junk food often deplete your metabolism swiftly.

Men mostly gain weight on the tummy, then the buttocks. Men look cylindrical when obese, while women look more triangular, pear-shaped, due to weight gain on the thighs.

**A SIX MONTH WEIGHT LOSS PLAN**

Begin with a 10 day detox program, as follows:

1. For the first one or two days, take in only warm ginger water, one cup every half hour, and nothing else at all. To make ginger water mix ¼ of a teaspoonful of dry ginger powder in five glasses of water, bring to the boil and let it cool. This assists in melting fat, improving metabolism, leading to a sense of lightness and improved energy.
2. For the next three days live on a mung and vegetable soup diet. To make the soup soak 1 cup (250 ml) of whole green mung overnight. Drain, add fresh water, salt and the spices of your choice. Cook in a pressure cooker with two cups (500 ml) of chopped vegetables—preferably leafy greens, squashes and pumpkins. Eat this soup warm, as many times a day as you want. You may drink tea once or twice a day rather than the soup.
3. For the following five days, add more vegetable to the mung, to make it thicker, along with mung patties or pancakes. Recommended vegetables include pumpkins, zucchinis (courgettes), kale, squashes, asparagus, leafy greens, broccoli, lauki, turai, tendli, and the padwal types of Indian vegetables.
4. After 10 days of this regime, measure yourself and see the difference!
5. From the 11th day onward, return to a normal diet, with the exclusion of fried, fermented and sour foods, wheat, red meat, cheese and yoghurt. Make sure that your diet is 60% vegetables, 35% protein (such as mung, lentils, tofu, fish, chicken, eggs), with a small quantity, up to 5% of carbohydrates such as rice,

millet or potatoes. It's fine to completely avoid carbohydrates. Follow this diet for next 6 months.

If you follow this detox diet for 10 days every month, or even every two months followed by diet as per point no. 5 on all other days, without doubt you will easily gain control over your weight, and look younger at the same time.

## LIFESTYLE

It is critically important to have a regular exercise routine. Spend one hour a day exercising your body in the following way: 20 minutes of yoga or Pilates; 30 minutes of cardiovascular exercise such as running, cycling, swimming, dancing, or aerobics; 10 minutes of weight training.

## PRANAYAMA

**Anulom vilom:** 10 minutes every day

**Kapalbhati:** 10 minutes every day

Focus on yoga postures for thighs, tummy, butts, and tyre reduction. Consult a yoga trainer for yoga postures like:

**Utkatasan** (chair pose): 5 times a day

**Hastapadasan** (standing forward bend): 5 times a day

**Suryanamaskar** (sun salutation): 5 times everyday including all 12 yoga postures.

Also do **Bhujangasan** (cobra pose), **Naukasan** (boat pose), and **Salabhasan** (locust pose) each 5 times a day.

## HOME REMEDY FOR MEN WHO WANT TO LOSE WEIGHT

This home remedy is amazing. If you take it regularly, it will help in both improving your metabolism and melting fat. You will lose weight easily.

### Horse gram/barley water

| | |
|---|---|
| Horse gram (kulathi) (or use barley) | 1 tblsp |
| Garcinia fruit (kokam) (optional) | 3 |
| Water | 2 cups (500 ml) |

Cook in a pressure cooker and filter.

Pour half of the mixture in one bowl and half in another. To one bowl of barley water, to drink in the morning, add and mix:

| | |
|---|---|
| Cumin powder | 1 tsp |
| Coriander powder | 1 tsp |
| Ajwain powder | ½ tsp |
| Asafoetida | 1 pinch |
| Dry ginger powder | ¼ tsp |
| Purified guggul (Commiphora wightii) powder | ½ tsp |

Make the mixture once more in the evening, using the remaining barley water, and drink it.

If you follow this remedy every day, you will easily lose two to three kilos a month. Many men have tried these remedies and lost up to 20 kilos in six to eight months. You won't believe how much more energetic, and youthful you will feel. You will also reduce metabolic problems like high cholesterol, high uric acid and high blood sugar. Of course, following diet is very important.

## AYUSHAKTI HERBAL REMEDIES

**Suhruday**: 2 tablets, twice a day—improves metabolism, while reducing sadness and stress.

**Mednil**: 3 tablets, 3 times a day—liquefies fats, which are eliminated through blood circulation.

## AYUSHAKTI'S DETOX PROGRAM

A profoundly effective way to control weight for both women men.

Detoxification at Ayushakti is an extremely powerful three to five week program which follows five steps; preparation, accumulation, elimination, lubrication and finally rejuvenation of the body. First, the body is prepared for the cleansing process by specific herbs and ghruts (medicated ghee). Then, using an anti-clog massage, all the toxins from everywhere in the body is pulled down to the digestive tract. Strong purgatives eliminate all toxins. These are visible in yellow mucous toxins in the stools. This process is very effective as toxins are removed even from the deepest tissue levels.

Detoxification helps to improve metabolism, reduces swelling, and removes the blocks of Ama toxins. This invigorates the circulation and bodily functions. You feel very light and refreshed due to the reduction in body weight.

This weight loss is usually maintained in a natural way, even after the detox is over, as your metabolism gets to work better.

*For Ayushakti supplements and clinics, see page iv.*

# 6. Diabetes

## Diabetes Type 2

I met a German doctor at my clinic in Munich. He was very surprised when I took his pulse reading and told him that he had very high blood sugar count of around 250, that he had weakness from some neuropathic changes in his legs, and his liver was fatty, because he had told me nothing about his condition. As an eminent neurosurgeon he was highly aware of the side effects in his body of daily insulin injections and oral tablets for his diabetes.

I promised him that he would be in control of his own blood sugar levels in 6 to 12 months. He was impressed and ready to do anything, so I began by dealing with his excess mucus, Ama, through focus on his diet and lifestyle, along with highly effective herbs for two months. Within that time he lost six kilos, and his daily insulin units were reduced from 20 to 15. He was very pleased with this, of course, and followed my advice to next do Panchkarma, deep detox, at the Ayushakti Clinic in India.

This process of removal of toxins from deep within the body brought great results for the doctor. He lost 12 kilos in just five weeks, and at the end of that time his sugar was being controlled naturally. He no longer needed daily insulin injections, and his need for allopathic tablets was greatly reduced.

After his Panchkarma I started him on a rejuvenation programme using Rasayana herbs, along with a special and lifestyle modifications to improve his pancreatic functions, reduce his fatty liver and the symptoms of neuropathic changes.

To this day he manages his blood sugar levels by the use of Ayushakti herbs, along with focus on diet and lifestyle.

## Guidance for Managing Blood Sugar Levels

### DIET

Healthy eating for diabetics includes:

- Limiting foods that are high in sugar
- Eating smaller portions, spread out over the day
- Being careful about when and how many carbohydrates you eat
- Eating a variety of whole-grain foods and vegetables every day
- Eating less fat
- Limiting your use of alcohol
- Using less salt

**Eat more**: Proteins like chickpeas, mung, lentils, masoor, mung dal, and soya bean products. Vegetables like spinach, leafy greens, dudhi (bottle gourd), turai, bhopla (white pumpkin), padwal (snake gourd), karela (bitter gourd), broccoli, cabbage, Brussel sprouts, zucchini, all leafy greens and all kinds of cooked vegetables are very good. Cereals like green millet, ragi, corn, kulit (horse gram), jwari and barley (jav).

**Note:** If you have a kidney problem, you may need more vegetables and less protein.

**Foods to avoid**: rice, potatoes, fruits, white flour, wheat, deep fried foods, red meat.

## Detox diet

- **First two days**—fasting with ginger water only
- **For the next 7 days** take only mung soup and vegetables
- **Next five days**, consume solid mung and vegetables
- Then come back to the **general diet**

This specific diet will help to remove blockages from the channels and toxins from the body, improves metabolism and help reduce blood sugar levels.

## LIFESTYLE

Walking daily for at least ½ hour is essential.

## HOME REMEDIES

### Powerful home remedies

Mix turmeric powder (haldi) ½ tsp + amala powder (Indian gooseberry) 1 tsp + fenugreek (methi) seeds powder ½ tsp in half glass of water and take daily in the morning on empty stomach.

### Herbal formula to reduce blood sugar

| | |
|---|---|
| Mamejava powder (Lenicostemma littrorale) | 100 g |
| Karella powder (bitter gourd) | 100 g |
| Gudmar (Gymnema sylvestre) powder | 100 g |
| Methi (fenugreek) powder | 50 g |
| Jambhoo beej (black plum) powder | 50 g |

Mix well and keep bottled. Take three tsp 2–3 times a day.

## AYUSHAKTI HERBAL REMEDIES

Effective herbal remedies to help remove blockages from the channels and insulin resistance.

**Sugarid tablet**: 2 tablets twice a day—removes blockages from the channels, improves metabolism. Improves physical energy. Rejuvenates body to balance sugar levels.

**Diabhar tablet**: 2 tablets twice a day—balances blood sugar levels. Promotes pancreas functions. Reduces fatigue, numbness, tiredness, dryness, weakness and giddiness related to diabetes and promotes physical energy and strength. Reduces sugar levels.

**Suhruday tablet**: 2 tablets twice a day—for stimulating metabolism and reducing stress.

## MARMA

Effective, safe and deep healing marma treatment for managing blood sugar. Kshipra marma is situated between the thumb and index finger as shown:

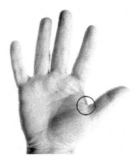

Method: Apply shunthi powder (dry ginger) on the marked area. Massage in circles with the thumb for five minutes on each hand, six times a day.

## PANCHKARMA AT AN AYUSHAKTI CLINIC

**Detoxification Panchkarma** includes five types of different detoxification treatments at deeper levels to eradicate the root cause of any poor health situation. Panchkarma regulates the metabolism and removes excess doshas and toxins which are the main reasons of metabolic blockages and insulin resistance. It not only stimulates the pancreas to function but also reduces insulin resistance thus reducing blood sugar naturally. Our experience is that this deep level detoxification keeps the blood sugar under control for 12 to 18 months naturally.

For high sugar levels, Virechan and Basti (medicated enema) is very important. First it prepares you by abhyanga, steam, and internal ghee to melt and bring the toxins to the digestive tract. On the tenth day, when the toxins come to the digestive tract, they are removed with strong purgation. This is followed by a herbal decoction, oils and daily enema given to extract air and mucous.

The next stage is the two-month rejuvenation program with special rejuvenation herbs, diet and lifestyle to improve pancreas functions, diminish fatty livers, the symptoms of neuropathic changes, and overall rejuvenation to the bodily channels.

By the end of the rejuvenation program, you may find that you can reduce, or even do without a high dosage of medication and control your sugar levels in a natural way.

This means that many people could control their sugar levels naturally only taking Ayushakti herbal formulations after detoxification.

**Virechan.** Internal cleansing of body through purgation therapy.

**Basti.** Medicated enema for further cleansing.

**Virechan and Basti have to be done with the guidance of an Ayushakti doctor.**


EASY TO COOK RECIPES

**Mung soup**

| | |
|---|---|
| Green mung beans | 1 cup |
| Onion, finely chopped | 1 |
| Fresh ginger grated or finely chopped | 1 knob |
| Safflower oil | 1 tblsp |
| Ground turmeric, cumin, coriander, fennel, pinch asafoetida, sea salt, black pepper | ½ tsp each |
| Bay leaf | 1 |
| Water | 6–8 cups |

Wash the mung beans. Soak for 30 minutes. Discard water and re-rinse. Heat safflower oil, add spices, onion and ginger. Sauté lightly, add mung beans and stir to coat for greater absorption of the spices. Add water and salt. Bring to boil and cook until the mung beans are completely soft. Add black pepper to taste. You can garnish with freshly chopped coriander.

**Vegetable soup**

| | |
|---|---|
| Vegetables—carrot, beans, white pumpkin, tendli (concinna), turai, snake gourd or zucchini | 2 cups |
| Water for cooking | 2 cups |
| Water for preparing the gravy | 1 cup |
| Ghee | 1 tblsp |
| Cumin | 1 tsp |
| Bay leaf | 1–2 |
| Curry leaves | 6 |
| Coriander seeds | 1 tsp |
| Salt | 1½ tsp |
| Turmeric | ½ tsp |
| Garlic paste | 1 tsp |
| Ginger paste | 1 tsp |
| Kokam water | ½ tsp |
| Green chilli (optional) | 1 |

Clean and chop all vegetables in 2–3 cm sized cubes. Add water and boil it in pressure cooker for 10–15 minutes or until vegetables become tender. Grind the cooked vegetables in a blender and add gradually the water. Then dilute the gravy by pouring the remained water. Heat the ghee in a deep saucepan. Reduce the fire to medium, add cumin, bay leaf, curry leaves and the coriander seeds. When the cumin is lightly brown, add ginger garlic paste, chilli. Then pour in the soup, add turmeric and salt. Finally stir in the kokam water and boil the soup for a few minutes.

**Pudla (pancake)**

| | |
|---|---|
| Mung dal flour | 1 cup |
| Water | as required |
| Safflower oil | |
| Salt | |
| Ginger | 1 tsp |
| Garlic paste | 1 tsp |
| Haldi (turmeric) | ¼ tsp |
| Red chilli powder | ¼ tsp |

In a bowl, mix mung dal and add enough water, whisk to runny batter consistency. Add ginger, garlic paste, turmeric and chilli powder. Mix well. Heat pan and add oil, spoon in batter evenly and cook pancake approximately two minutes on each side until golden. Serve with green chutney.

**Note:** You can also use soaked and grinded green mung in place of mung dal flour. Also add garam masala, green chilli etc. to taste.

## QUICK CHECKLIST FOR MANAGING YOUR BLOOD SUGAR LEVELS

- Eat meals at regular intervals and do not overeat.
- Walk for at least ½ hour daily—this very important
- If you notice dryness in your mouth, along with thirst, numbness, fatigue, pain in muscles, or frequent urination, consult your physician.
- Do not smoke. Smoking leads to heart disease and poor circulation
- Get good sleep every night
- Check your blood sugar levels regularly
- Check your weight regularly and maintain ideal body weight

- Reduce your intake of alcohol
- Avoid rice, potatoes, and fruits completely
- Make chapattis with 75% chickpea flour and 25% wheat instead of full wheat
- Avoid bread and pasta, eat mung or chickpea pancakes or tofu, corn, and millet pasta
- 70% of your diet should be vegetables.

*For Ayushakti supplements and clinics, see page iv.*

# 7. Reducing High Cholesterol

High cholesterol is an epidemic in our society. By the age of 45 people often begin to take anti-cholesterol tablets, which have long term side-effects, gastritis and muscle wasting for example, which makes people feel very weak. We take this medication because of our fear of the heart problems it may cause.

But all this is not necessary. It's completely possible to control cholesterol naturally. This is because high cholesterol is a consequence of low metabolism, which leads to Ama in the blood, so when you activate your metabolism, naturally your body stops producing excess cholesterol.

This is the story of John from the USA, who had already had very high cholesterol for three years by the age of 35. He'd tried everything he could to change his diet: no butter, no oils, taking flax seeds, olive oil—but nothing reduced his cholesterol level.

When I met him in New York I told him that first of all he needed to do Panchkarma at the Ayushakti Clinic, because this would increase his metabolism very quickly. After a full five week Panchkarma in India his cholesterol became normal. When he went home his doctors told him to keep on doing what you are doing now.

However, if you don't have a chronic problem or can't manage a full Panchkarma you can manage it through diet and detox. For seven days every month eat only mung and vegetable soup, which over time will activate your metabolism,

Along with this diet, John took a powder made from psyllium husk (isabgol) and fenugreek (methi) two tablespoons twice a day for six months, and his cholesterol became completely normal. After that time, if his cholesterol level rose, he would fast and take this powder again. In this way he has handled his cholesterol levels for the last ten years

## What is Good and Bad cholesterol?

Total cholesterol comprises of HDL, LDL, (high- and low-density lipoproteins) and triglycerides.

HDL is a good cholesterol, and higher HDL protects you against heart problems. So your total cholesterol should be 200 mg/dl. HDL should be at least 20% to 30%. So even if cholesterol is slightly higher with HDL 60 mg/dl, you should not worry about heart problems. Focus on increasing your good cholesterol and keep triglycerides under control.

### DIET

Avoid an Ama-reducing diet and saturated fat.

Totally avoid all fatty food, oily food, spicy items and red meat in your diet. Do not eat white rice, white sugar, oils such as groundnut oil, mustard oil, refined foods, and milk products because these are heavy to digest.

Eat food high in fibre for immediate cholesterol reduction, for example oatmeal, roti, or bread made of red and white millets and ragi or rye, for breakfast.

For lunch, eat more vegetables, salads, soups, up to 60% of your meal, and 30 per cent as proteins like mung, mung dal, green vegetables etc.

For dinner, have very light food like mung pancake, fruits, jwari roti or corn, quinoa, pasta or bread, proteins like lentils, legumes, tofu, or lean meat like fish and chicken, and dal.

Eat fresh leaves of fenugreek, amaranth, argul, kale, or spinach at least 100 g per day. Olive oil is the best oil to use, or a combination of flax seed and olive oil, or flax seed and soya bean oil.

## LIFESTYLE

- Walk for at least 45 minutes every day.
- Practise Pranayama (Anulom Vilom Pranayama) and meditation to relieve stress
- Avoid smoking and alcohol.

## HOME REMEDIES

**1.**

Take 1 to 2 tblsp flax seeds (alsi) powder.

1 tsp of fenugreek powder

1 tblsp of psilium husk powder

Mix together and drink with water twice a day.

**2.**

Take 2 to 3 cloves of garlic daily. It reduces harmful cholesterol in the blood, frees up the arteries and improves blood circulation.

**3.**

1 tsp of flaxseed oil: drink it on empty stomach to increase good cholesterol.

## AYUSHAKTI HERBAL REMEDIES

**Cholestrin** powder: 2 tsp twice a day

## MARMA

Apply ghee on the temples and soles of the feet and massage for five minutes daily to reduce stress; recommended before sleeping.

## PANCHKARMA AT AN AYUSHAKTI CLINIC

If the cholesterol level is very high, then a super detox Panchkarma for 4–5 weeks greatly helps to reduce the cholesterol levels by removing the excess fat and toxins accumulated in the body. The super detox Panchkarma also reduces the risk of heart problems and obesity.

*For Ayushakti supplements and clinics, see page iv.*

# 8. Balancing High Blood Pressure

High blood pressure is a result of high Ama and Pitta in the blood. Both are kinds of mucus; Pitta is liquid and hot, Ama is simply toxic. Pitta we need in balance, Ama we don't need or want at all. After years of high pita and Ama getting deposited into the bloodstream, the blood volume itself increases. Sometimes this toxic mucus accumulates in the form of plaque in the arteries, and because of this the circulation becomes blocked. It works in the same way that when a pipe gets blocked it begins to swell, nothing can pass through it easily and pressure increases. When there are deposits in the arteries and the blood volume has increased, it leads to high blood pressure. The key solution for this is to remove the Pitta toxins through a tailored detox process.

A good example is Satyapriya, from the UK. She was in India on a spiritual retreat, and came to me for a consultation. When I took her blood pressure it gave me high blood pressure! She told me she didn't want to take allopathic medicine, so I told her to come to the clinic and do a special seven day detox. I gave her only mung soup and vegetables for seven days, with the instructions that when she went home, she should eat 70% vegetables, 20% mung and 10% protein, and hardly any carbohydrates, for six months. This diet dissolves the mucus which forms blockages in the arteries. At the clinic, together with this diet, we gave her specific purgations to remove hot Pitta toxins from the blood, and herbs to calm her hypertension, along with Shirodhara and specific marma points she could do at home.

This whole process of toxin dissolving and removal, by following a diet that reduced Ama and mucus and improved circulation, together with taking calming herbs, led to her blood pressure returning to normal—and my blood pressure too! It took one year, and now she's just fine, and doesn't need any treatment at all.

## How to Calm High Blood Pressure

### Diet

Diet should be low calcium, and Ama- and Pitta-reducing. Coffee can create temporary spike in blood pressure. Canned foods and pizza contain high sodium which increases Ama.

**Avoid:** Deep fried, spicy, fatty, salty, sour, pungent food. Avoid wheat, red meat, pickles and excess intake of yogurt, tomato, fermented food and alcohol. Also avoid processed deli meats, as they are sodium bombs (mostly they are preserved using high sodium).

**Eat more**: Foods like mung, lentils, zucchini and squashes, leafy vegetables, pumpkin, millet, red rice, rye, spelt, yellow dal and tofu; plenty of vegetables and protein is good.

Watermelon, banana, dark chocolate (specially pure cocoa powder), sunflower seeds (unsalted), whole grain instead of refined food, spinach, sweet potatoes, beans like chickpeas, kidney beans, and blueberries are best in regulating blood pressure.

## LIFESTYLE

- Take proper rest, and avoid frequent late nights
- Yoga, meditation, walking and light exercise are calming and beneficial
- Practice Pranayama and Anulom Vilom
- Learn to diminish the effects of tension, anxiety, and anger, perhaps through meditation.
- Avoid over-exertion
- Avoid exposure to extreme heat or cold
- Avoid suppression of natural urges like sneezing, coughing, burping etc.

## HOME REMEDIES

### High blood pressure due to tension

**1.**

| | |
|---|---|
| Cinnamon powder | ¼ tsp |
| Jaifal | 1 pinch |
| Mixture ginger, black pepper, long pepper powders | ¼ tsp |
| Gotucola powder | 1 tsp |
| Sarpagandha powder | 1 tsp |

Mix all in half glass of water and drink twice a day

**2.**

White pumpkin (English marrow) juice daily

**3.**

Barley water, three times a day. (Pressure-cook and filter 1 tblsp of barley and 4 glasses of water, and reduce it by half.)

| | |
|---|---|
| Barley water | ½ of the amount prepared |
| Cumin powder | 1 tsp |
| Coriander powder | 1 tsp |
| Rose petals | 1 heads |
| Cardamom | 2 tsp |
| Fennel seed powder | 1 tsp |
| Asafoetida | 1 pinch |

Mix well and drink twice daily.

## AYUSHAKTI HERBAL REMEDY

**Raktashanti**: 2 tablets twice a day. This formula helps to control high blood pressure, improve circulation, and reduce the stress and anxiety related to high blood pressure. Regular use of **Raktashanti** helps to reduce blood pressure.

**Suhruday**: 2 tablets twice a day. Helps to reduce stress, anxiety, improves blood circulation, and heart functions.

## Marma

### Marma points to reduce high blood pressure

**1.**

Apply ghee to the temples, and to the centre of the head. Massage gently for five minutes.

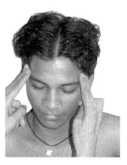

**Fig. 1**

**2.**

Apply ghee on the soles of the feet and massage with a kasa vati (bronze bowl).

**3.**

Press the marma points located in the centre of the sole as shown in figures 2 and 3. These points should be pressed continuously in sets of six while relaxing.

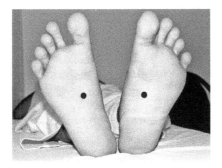

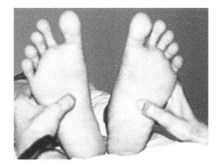

**Fig. 2**                    **Fig. 3**

**4.**

Apply ghee to the navel, the temporal areas and on the top of the head.

Press the marma points located on the temples, as shown in figure 1 (above), with your index and middle finger. With gentle pressure slide the fingers down through the temple region, six times. Press this marma point located on the forehead between the eyes as shown in figure 4, with your right thumb, six times.

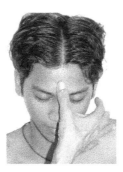

**Fig. 4**

**5.**

Apply ghee to the marma point located between the eyes. Press this point with the right thumb as shown in figure 4 (above); rock the thumb's pad from tip down, six times. Allow the patient to remain in this state of deep relaxation for three minutes and while continuously pressing this marma point, repeat in a very soft voice: 'Day by day I become healthy, full of energy and dynamic. My blood pressure becomes completely normal.'

Repeat this marma exercise as frequently as needed, or until blood pressure becomes normal. Do this every day. Regular use of marma will help to reduce blood pressure.

## Panchkarma

### Ayushakti clinic treatments

Shirodhara and heartdhara are very effective in reducing (lowering) high blood pressure. Shirodhara and heartdhara should be done with the help of a qualified Ayurvedic Vaidhya.

### Shirodhara

Mix one teaspoon of ghee in half glass of warm milk. Lay down and pour this lukewarm liquid continuously in a thin stream on the third eye point (bindi point) for 20 minutes. Reheat the liquid to keep the warm temperature till end of the process.

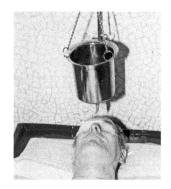

# Raising Low Blood Pressure

Low blood pressure can be due to low circulation, often due to lower iron in blood. It can create lots of tiredness and dizziness.

**HOME REMEDIES**

**1.**

| | |
|---|---|
| Pipar longum root (pippali root) | ¼ tsp |
| Ginger powder | ¼ tsp |
| Black pepper powder | ¼ tsp |
| Milk | ½ cup |
| Water | ½ cup |

Mix well and drink after every 2–3 hours.

**2.**

| | |
|---|---|
| Dates | 4 |
| Almonds | 4 |
| Fennel | 1 tsp |
| Cardamom | 2 |
| Ghee | 1 tsp |
| Jaggery | 1 tsp |
| Ginger powder | ¼ tsp |

Blend into a paste and eat in the morning on an empty stomach.

## MARMA

This Marma helps to create conscious, instant energy.

Press the marma point located at the base of the nose between the nostrils, as shown. Press this point with your index finger six times, six times a day.

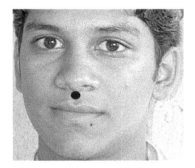

## Ayushakti herbal remedies

**Suhruday**: 2 tablets twice a day—creates energy, improves blood circulation, and balances blood pressure.

**Jeevanrakshak**: 2 tablets twice a day—instantly raises blood pressure and reduces anxiety and panic feeling.

*For Ayushakti supplements and clinics, see page iv.*

# 9.   Coughs and Colds

## Introduction

Breathing is a critically important process in our bodies; with the inhale it brings oxygen into the body, with the exhale it removes carbon dioxide. Life itself is dependent on the breath. For this reason, whenever we are exposed to viruses, bacteria or dust particles through the breath, the immune system becomes hyperactive immediately, to remove them from the body.

The immune system responds in the form of mucus within the respiratory system, which dissolves the foreign particles within it, then expels them through coughs and colds. This means they are in fact a defence mechanism which keeps our respiration system clear.

This makes coughs and colds sound simple and useful, but for those who suffer from them over a long period of time, life can be miserable. Work, socializing, outdoor activities, the quality of life itself suffers. We need to handle this problem in the best way possible.

**Ayushakti** specializes in chronic and acute colds, asthma and immune deficiency syndromes. We have treated thousands of people around the world using a combination of conscious diet, home remedies and herbs, which I will share with you below.

The most common causes of respiratory problems are:

- Exposure to bacterial or viral infections.
- Allergies to dust, fungal particles, fumes, certain foods etc.
- Smoker's syndrome – people who smoke cough because of the irritating effect of the smoke and damage it causes to the cells of respiratory tract.
- Long term exposure to irritating factors such as smoke, dust, other pollutants etc.
- A low immune response in the body.

We will be discussing the four commonly seen ailments seen in this category:

1. Common viral coughs
2. Cold, nasal congestions and sinusitis
3. Chronic coughs, throat infections and irritations, ear infections
4. Allergic breathlessness & bronchitis

# Common Viral Cough

### Introduction

A cough is a sudden explosive movement of air to clear material from respiratory airways. It helps to protect the lungs from foreign particles. Coughing can bring up phlegm, a mixture of mucus, debris and cells. If it becomes severe and chronic it can result in shortness of breath, hoarseness, dizziness and wheezing. Viral coughs are highly contagious, and spread quickly in any social group.

- Coughing, hoarseness of voice
- Irritation in the throat
- Fatigue and body aches
- A cold, if the infection has spread to the nose

Colds usually heal themselves within seven days, whether you take medication or not. Anything you take to suppress a cough is useless. In fact, suppression dries up the cough, leaving a dry cough which can last for months.

Mucus and coughing play an important role in clearing infections and particles in the respiratory system. The best thing we can do is to help our system to liquefy and expel the mucus easily, diminishing the seven days of inconvenience and suffering.

Let me share with you a very safe and effective home remedy. This helps clear the congestion and expel the mucus.

### Home remedy

| | |
|---|---|
| Fresh ginger juice | ¼ tsp |
| Turmeric powder | ¼ tsp |
| Garlic juice | ¼ tsp |
| Fresh basil leaf juice | ½ tsp |
| Honey | 2 tsp |
| Black pepper powder | 1 pinch |

Mix all the ingredients well. Keep it refrigerated if you are making a large quantity and wish to use again, then bring it to room temperature before using. Take 1½ teaspoons of this mixture four times a day. Children can safely take this cough mixture.

## DIET, AND LIFESTYLE PLAN FOR COUGHS, COLDS, BREATHLESSNESS AND ALLERGIES

### Foods to avoid

Foods such as wheat, refined white flour, meat (especially red meat), refined sugar, deep fried foods. These foods decrease the digestive fire (Agni) and produce mucus (kapha) and toxins (Ama).

All sweet fruits, such as apples, pears, apricots, cherries, plums, sweet berries, fresh figs and dates, mangoes, papayas, water melons and pomegranates, which are very cold in energy & produce excessive mucus.

Milk and milk products are also mucus producing so should be best avoided.

Ice cold foods and drinks are immediate 'killers 'of the digestive fire. They also produce excess mucus.

### Foods to enjoy

Cooked vegetables such as pumpkin (kaddu), squashes, marrow, courgette, Ivy Gourd/ Gentleman's Toes (Tendli), spinach (Palak),fenugreek leaves (Methi), French beans, bottle gourds(Dudhi), ridge gourds (Turai), snake gourd (Padwal), smooth gourd (Galka), mange-tout, asparagus, fennel, dill leaves, Swiss chord, sweet corn, onions, carrots, parsnips beetroot, celery, chicory and leeks. Potatoes should only be eaten occasionally, with their skin.

Pulses are an essential part of a healthy diet. Mung and split Mung beans (green gram), Tuvar Dal (pigeon peas) and Masoor Dal (red lentils) are easy to digest, balancing and nourishing to the body. To get the full value from pulses they should be eaten along with grains (especially rice).

Grains including rice, oat, rye, maize (makai), millets (jawar, bajra nachani) amaranth (rajigira), quinoa, kamut, spelt, polenta; basically everything other than wheat. Flours made from the above grains and also from potatoes and buckwheat are excellent substitutes for 'normal 'flour.

Dried fruits like apricots and dates, and nuts like almonds, walnuts, pistachio, hazel nuts can be eaten.

One can enjoy white meat like chicken, turkey, and fish (fresh water) occasionally, if you are used to eating non-vegetarian food.

You can replace dairy milk with almond milk, rice milk, soya milk or oat milk.

This diet improves our defence mechanism.

## LIFESTYLE

- Do not smoke.
- Avoid exposure to cold, winds, dust, fumes and other pollutants, or cover your head, ears and nose to protect yourself from their effect.
- Give your vocal cords a rest by talking less.
- Drink warm water, not cold, throughout the day.
- Drink hot tea made of tulsi, ginger and mint leaves.

## YOGA AND EXERCISE

Exercise and practice yoga as a daily routine, as it will improve and maintain the oxygen carrying capacity of the blood.

Pranayam plays a very important role in getting relief from coughs and colds. Practice the yogic breathing techniques of Bhastrika, Kapalbhati and Ujjayi Pranayamas, etc. (details given below) for wet coughs do all every morning for 15 to 20 minutes, and do Shitali and Sitkari for dry coughs 5 to 10 times.

Bhastrika pranayam: 5 times

Kapalbhati: 10 minutes

Anulom vilom: 10 minutes

Ujjayi pranayam: 5 times

Shitali and Sitkari pranayam: each 5 to 10 times

Also do all these neck-related exercises:

- Turn your neck right to left and left to right for 10 times
- Turn your neck up and down 10 times
- Turn neck clockwise 5 times
- Do anti clock rotation of neck 5 times

Omkar (a kind of pranayam): repeat 5 times back to back.

Take a long breath as much you can and while exhaling say 'om'. O for a longer time and M for a shorter time.

Jalneti: do once


## RECOMMENDED AYUSHAKTI HERBAL REMEDIES

**Divyaswas jivan**: 1 tablet 3 times a day—effectively stops runny nose and cough

**Kaphano syrup**: 2 teaspoon (small spoon) twice a day—expels cough smoothly

**D-Vyro**: 1 tablet twice a day for immune boosting

These herbs have been proven to be effective for more than 27 years. They soothe sore throats and deal with coughs, liquefying and expelling mucus and clearing congestion.

# Allergic Colds, Nasal Congestion and Sinusitis

## Introduction

Cough and colds are not only caused by infection but also by allergies. Exposure to grass, weeds, tree pollen, dust mites, petrol fumes, perfume sprays, cat or dog hairs, as well as foods such as milk or peanuts can create a strong histamine reaction. This is an immunological response in the form of massive mucus generation, which removes allergic particles.

The body response to the common cold is similar. It is our immune response to both infection and allergic particles.

## Symptoms

- repeated sneezing
- a runny nose followed by congestion and blocked sinus
- nasal blockage with difficulty in breathing and subsequent wheezing
- headaches, which may be followed by fever

It is possible to identify the cause of the cold by examining the sputum (the mucus). Yellowish, greenish or brownish mucus indicates bacterial infection; clear and sticky mucus indicates a food or atmospheric allergy.

Suppression of the mucus with medication causes irritation and continued congestion. The best solution is to support our body by making the immune system strong along with liquefying the mucus to aid its expulsion.

Dealing with the occasional cold, say every 4-6 months is no problem. Problems arise when allergic colds come almost daily or weekly. The condition then turns into recurrent chronic sinusitis, where the sinuses (the spaces within the bones in the head) become blocked due to infective mucus.

**Ayushakti** has successfully helped many such people with the help of herbs. These herbs build and strengthen the immune system, liquefy mucus, ease breathing. Congestion is cleared at its root, so it does not return easily.

## HOME REMEDY

### 1.

### Herbal tea

| | |
|---|---|
| Fresh ginger crushed | ½ tsp |
| Basil leaves crushed | 12 |
| Black pepper crushed | 3 |
| Cardamom, crushed | 3 |
| Mint leaves, crushed | 5 |
| Cinnamon, crushed | ½ inch |
| Water | 1¼ cup |
| Honey | 1 tblsp |

Bring water to the boil then add all the ingredients except the honey. Boil the mixture for one minute, keeping it covered. Remove from the heat and cover the vessel with a lid for 5 minutes. Filter and add the honey.

This warm tea should be taken 3 to 4 times a day.

You can also use the cough recipes which I have showed you previously.

**2.**

**Ajwain** (carom seeds) or wild celery seeds  2 tsp

Roast the ajwain (carom) seeds on a griddle. Inhale the fumes until the smell of ajwain seeds fades, then begin the process again with fresh seeds. Inhale the ajwain seed fumes in this way for five minutes.

**3.**

| | |
|---|---|
| Garlic juice | ¼ tsp |
| Water | 2 tsp |

Lie down and insert ½ teaspoon of this mixture into each nostril twice a day. It burns, but cuts through congestion, while the garlic kills off any bacterial infection.

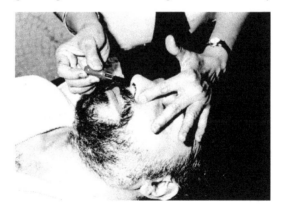

## DIET

Follow the diet as recommended earlier.

## Recommended Ayushakti herbal remedies

**Asthloc**: 2 tablets twice a day—clears congestion and breathlessness

**D-Vyro**: 2 tablets twice a day—improves immune system

## Yoga and exercise

As described earlier.

# Chronic Coughs, Throat Irritations and Ear Infections

## Introduction

Sometimes coughs and throat infections do not clear up completely. Mucus can then remain in the nose and sinus areas. This can lead to a chronic cough, throat irritations and ear infections. Recurrent occurrence of the following symptoms is a sign of lowered immunity.

- Constant coughing, with or without mucus
- Irritation and redness of throat
- Hoarseness in the voice
- Earache and itching in the ear
- Headaches, a sense of malaise
- Reduced sense of both smell and hearing

**Ayushakti** has successfully cured many such chronic cases, giving sufferers a new lease of life. The following case study demonstrates its effectiveness.

When I took part in a radio show in Los Angeles 10 years ago, a Mrs Jain called and told me of her problem. More than two months previously she had taken antibiotics which cleared her throat infection, but her congestion remained. During the night her nose became completely blocked, and she had trouble breathing for up to two hours. I recommended the powerful home remedy you can see below. This remedy activated her digestion, diminished the production of mucus and helped boost her immune system. After just one week she called to say that her congestion had been much reduced in just three days, and after that one week she could breathe easily.

## DIET

Follow the diet as described earlier.

## HOME REMEDIES

**1.**

| | |
|---|---|
| Fresh basil (Tulsi) leaves | 10 |
| Black peppers (whole) | 2 |

Chew them together on an empty stomach in the morning. When half chewed, swallow the mixture with water. Repeat this in the evening and once more at night before going to bed.

**2.**

At night put 2-4 drops of warm castor oil in each nostril before going to sleep.

**3.**

Mix the following ingredients to make a pill to suck 3 to 6 times a day.

| | |
|---|---|
| Turmeric powder | ¼ tsp |
| Liquorice powder | ¼ tsp |
| Honey | enough to make a pill |

### AYUSHAKTI HERBAL REMEDIES

**Asthaloc**: 2 tablets twice a day—clears congestion and improves breathlessness

**D-Vyro**: 2 tablets twice a day—boost immune system

**Kaphano syrup**: 1 tsp—lubricates cough

**Antisepta lozenges**: antiseptic for the throat

# Allergic Breathlessness Bronchitis

## Introduction

It is clear to us all that a clear pathway for air to reach into our lungs, bringing essential oxygen to our blood and tissues is essential for life. When the airways are inflamed or blocked by bronchitis or asthma this access is reduced, with clear consequences, so they need to be dealt with effectively.

Acute bronchitis is an inflammation of the lining of the airways caused by viral or bacterial infection. It usually resolves itself. Chronic bronchitis can be triggered by long-term exposure to irritants such as tobacco, smoke, dust or chemicals.

Asthma is an inflammatory condition that leads to a tightening of the muscles around the airways. This leads to consequent swelling and narrowing, with a restriction of airflow.

## Comparison of symptoms

**Bronchitis**

- Cough
- Production of mucus (sputum): clear, gray or green
- Slight fever and chills and fatigue.
- Chest discomfort

**Asthma**

- Coughing especially at night
- Sleepless nights
- Wheezing
- Shortness of breath/ breathlessness
- Weakness after exercise
- Chest tightness, pressure and pain

Suppressing asthma attacks by dilating the airways is neither effective enough nor long lasting. To be truly effective treatment should lead to:

- Reduction in inflammation of airways, leading to a reduction of blockages in entire passageway
- Control over the contraction of chest muscles
- Melting of the mucus lodged in airways
- Improvement in overall immunity

**Ayushakti** has helped many people across the world with bronchitis and breathlessness. These people now sleep without breathlessness and congestion. With the improvement of their lung function and immunity their quality of life is greatly improved.

## YOGA AND EXERCISE

As described earlier.

## ASTHMA MUDRA

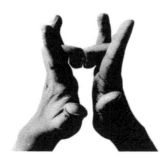

Fold the middle finger of both your hands so that their fingernails are positioned as touching each other. Keep the other fingers of both the hands straight and extended as much as possible. This is very effective for preventing asthma attacks.

## BRONCHIAL MUDRA

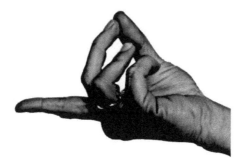

Place your little finger at the bottom of the thumb and the ring finger on the upper thumb joint. Now, place the middle finger on the pad of the thumb and likewise expand your index finger. Make use of this mudra for at least 4-6 minutes.

## NASYA TREATMENT FOR FASTER RELIEF OF BLOCKED NOSE OR SINUS

Put one drop of garlic juice in both nostrils. This will burn slightly inside the nose, but do not worry.

## HOME REMEDY

**1.**

Keep drinking warm ginger water throughout the day instead of regular water (one teaspoon ginger powder mixed in 5 glasses of water, bring to the boil then drink warm).

**2.**

For clearing congestion, melting and naturally expelling of the thick mucus for easy breathing:

| | |
|---|---|
| Cinnamon | approx. ½ inch stick (or use ¼ tsp powdered) |
| Water | 1¼ cup |
| Fresh ginger, crushed | ½ tsp |
| Basil leaves, crushed | 12 leaves |
| Black pepper, crushed | 3 peppercorns |
| Cardamom crushed | 3 seeds |
| Mint leaves crushed | 10 leaves |
| Honey | 1 tbspn |

Heat the water; when it begins to boil, add all the crushed ingredients except the honey. Boil the mixture for 2-3 minutes, keeping it covered. Switch off the heat, and cover the vessel with a lid for 5 minutes, then filter and add the honey. Mix well.

This warm tea should be taken 3 to 4 times a day.

**3.**

| | |
|---|---|
| Liquorice powder | 1 tsp |
| Vasa powder | 1 tsp |
| Kantakari powder | 1 tsp |

Mix all powder and take with ½ glass of water twice a day.

## RECOMMENDED AYUSHAKTI HERBAL REMEDIES

**Swasavin Asthaloc**: 2 tablets twice a day—for relieving breathlessness

**Kaphno syrup**: 2 teaspoons twice a day—for clearing the congestion

**D-Vyro**: 2 tablets twice a day—for improving the immune system

*For Ayushakti supplements and clinics, see page iv.*

# 10. Hair Loss and Hair Care

If you want to understand the way your hair grows, think of the plants in a garden. How they grow depends entirely on what is happening with their roots. The same is true for your hair. To understand and fix hair loss, we must deal with their roots, or follicles, and how they work.

Hair follicles grow in three natural phases:

**Anagen**: the growth phase; typically 1 centimetre every 28 days

**Catagen**: the follicle rests; no growth

**Telogen:** the hair falls out

According to Ayurveda, your hair is a by-product of bone tissue. Your bones produce BMP (bone morphogenetic protein) which nourishes the hair follicles internally and supports hair growth. It is normal for hairs to fall out, balanced by fresh hairs replacing them. If your nourishment of essentials such as protein and calcium are reduced, the anagen, growth stage, is not productive. So your hair which is lost is not replaced. This results in hair thinning and loss.

**The most common causes of hair loss**

- Excessive heat
- Autoimmune disorders
- Slow metabolism
- Loss of calcium in the body
- Stress
- Hormonal changes
- Thyroid imbalance
- Menopause
- Lack of sleep
- Adverse effects of therapies such as chemotherapy and radiation.

At **Ayushakti** we specialise in hair thinning and loss . We have successfully treated many thousands of people, all around the world. In the following sections I will share with you what I know works so well, from long experience. The methods use diet, home remedies and herbs, which are natural and without side-effects.

Specific problems we will cover:

- Hair loss due to inner heat or lack of nutrients
- Male pattern, U-shape baldness
- Hairline thinning in females
- Alopecia areata

If you have one of these problems, you will know the effects well. Hair loss can affect your life profoundly. People who suffer from hair loss can feel depressed. They can lose confidence in their personal and professional lives. For these reasons it is essential to deal with the problem of losing hair.

# Hair Loss due to Excess Internal Heat or Lack of Nutrients

Between the ages of 20 to 35 is the time of Pitta in our lives. This means we typically feel such qualities as ambition, creativity or aggression. You can also feel heat within the head. Many of us use protein oils, shampoos and conditioners to nourish the hair roots, but find that nothing works when hair loss begins.

After the age of 35 both women and men begin depletion of calcium from the bones. Women also lose a lot of calcium post delivery, and more from 40 to 50 years old, due to menopausal changes.

According to both Ayurveda and modern science, hair is a by-product of bone tissue. Bones themselves are nourished by calcium. BMP, which I mentioned above, nourishes your hair follicles and helps hair to grow. This is where the solution to hair loss lies.

The cause of these conditions lies in excess stress, aggravated Vata (air) and excessive internal heat. These cause a tightness of the scalp. In turn this leads to constricted arteries in the hair roots, which denies nutrients to the follicles.

### HOME REMEDIES

**1.**

A glass of pomegranate, grape, or amla (emblic fruit) juice, mixed with ½ tsp. of turmeric, which reduces heat and improves the blood supply to the hair root.

**2.**

1 tblsp of sesame seeds—a good source of natural calcium

**3.**

5 almonds or 5 walnuts—another source of calcium

## LIFESTYLE

Reducing stress is important in controlling hair loss—practice: pranayama, meditation, anulom vilom.

Yoga postures like Halasana (plough) and Sarvangasana (bridge) help to improve blood flow in the scalp.

Deep sleep is necessary: see the sleep section of this book.

## EFFECTIVE DIET GUIDELINES

**Avoid**: sour or fermented foods, wheat products and acidic foods. Add lots of calcium rich foods such as milk, sesame seeds—2 tblsp daily, spinach—1 cup daily, rajgira (amaranth)—100 g daily. This both nourishes the hair and reduces inner heat.

Add protein rich food such as almonds, pistachios, flax seeds, sesame seeds, pumpkin seeds, mung beans, corn, rice, oats, soybeans, navy, white, French and kidney beans, broccoli, cabbage, chick peas, coconut, avocado, walnuts, and wheat germ oil.

## GENERAL DIET TO SUPPORT HAIR GROWTH

**Avoid:** wheat, sour, fermented and Pitta-increasing food, sugar. Reduce high glycaemic carbohydrate foods such as rice and potatoes.

**Eat more:** High protein foods such as : milk, soya milk, tofu, cheese (low-fat mozzarella and cottage cheese), low fat paneer. Seeds such as pumpkin, squash, flax, sesame and watermelon. Nuts such as peanuts, almonds, and pistachios. Bran (corn, brown rice, oat), mung and soy beans, lentils, navy, white, French and kidney beans, broccoli, cabbage, chick peas.

**High fibre foods:** fortified cereals, toasted wheat germ, oatmeal, figs, apricots, coconut, lima beans, avocado, dates, raspberries. Soy foods. Vegetable oils such as, coconut oil, sunflower oil, olive oil, flax seed oil, walnut oil, rice bran oil, wheat germ oil. For non vegetarians: fish such as tuna and salmon, eggs (especially the whites), oysters, white meat. Foods rich in Beta Sitosterol, which supports hair growth: bananas, oranges, legumes, brown rice, nuts, pumpkin and sesame seeds.

## HERBS

**Ayushakti's Sukesha (tablets)** has been proven to be effective for more than 27 years. It effectively stops hair loss and promotes hair growth, by reducing inner heat and increasing BMP (see above).

# Male Pattern Baldness (U-shaped)

This type of hair loss is most common in males. It is usually related to genes & male sex hormones. It usually follows a pattern of a receding hairline followed by the hair thinning on the crown.

## Causes

Hormonal imbalance, low metabolism and inner heat are the main factors responsible. Low SHBG and high free testosterone levels lead to hair loss and diminished libido in men.

GF (growth factor) is responsible for hair growth in men. Obesity reduces GF and SHBG. A high protein and low carbohydrate diet increases GF.

Due to high inner heat and low metabolism, blood vessels to the follicles are constricted.

## Symptoms

Thinning of hair at the crown and front. Increased beard growth along with an increase in weight and acidity. Typical pattern of male baldness begins with the hairline gradually moving backwards, forming an 'M' shape. Eventually the hair becomes finer, thinner, and shorter and creates a 'U' shaped pattern of hair around the sides and back of the head.

### HOME REMEDIES

Pomegranate juice, ½ cup, 1 banana, ½ cup sweet grape juice, blend and drink daily.

### LIFESTYLE

Exercise in the following way:

Warm up for 3 minutes, for example running on a treadmill at 4 to 5 km/hr for 30-60 seconds, followed by fast vigorous exercise — running at 6 to 8 km for 2 minutes or more. Recover slowly by slowing down to 4 km/hr for 90 seconds. Repeat this sequence 7 times.

Reduce stress by practising Pranayama, meditation, and Anulom Vilom.

Deep sleep is vital. (see the sleep section of this book)

## MARMA

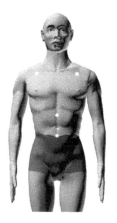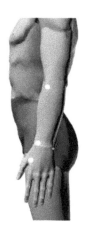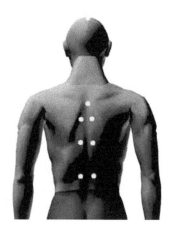

Pressing the points marked by the yellow dots can help restore hair growth. It is not necessary to use all these points; just using one or two of them when you have a free hands can really help. It is important to drink lots of warm water after massaging in this way. this helps to clear toxins from your body.

## DIET

The recommended general hair loss diet as above.

## HERBS

**Ayushakti's Sukesha** (tablets) is highly recommended and effective. It has been proven over time to reduce stop hair loss and promote hair growth. It reduces inner heat and increases BMP.

# Hairline Thinning in Women

As I have told you above, your hair growth comes in three phases. When your hair naturally falls out, it is replaced by new growth. When the new growth does not occur, the hairline will thin out, with a band-like pattern of hair loss. After time the follicles with cease to be active. Women are most likely to suffer from this condition after menopause, and is connected to hormonal changes.

The only solution for this is to control the ratio of hair fall and stimulate the new hair growth. Ayurveda's hair care solutions like hair growth and preventing hair fall and fighting against dandruff are the scientific ways for this.

## Reasons

- Polycystic Ovarian Syndrome (PCOS)
- Hormonal changes
- High stress
- Bearing many children
- Lack of sleep
- Lack of exercise
- Hypertension
- Divorce may cause hormonal changes and hairline thinning in women

The blood vessels leading to the hair follicles become constricted, due to high inner heat, hormonal imbalance and low metabolism. The denial of nutrients lead to hair loss and thinning of the hairline.

## Symptoms

- Hairline widening
- Temporary hair loss
- Dry scalp
- Scalp allergies, with itching and boils

### HOME REMEDIES

Take all below ingredients in powder form

| | |
|---|---|
| Yashtimadhu (liquorice) | 1 tsp |
| Jeera (cumin seeds) | 1 tsp |
| Ajwain (carom seeds) | ¼ tsp |
| Hing (asafoetida) | 1 pinch |
| Black salt | ½ tsp |
| Sauf (fennel seed) | ½ tsp |
| Ashok (bark of Ashok tree) | ½ tsp |

Mix all the powders together and drink with half a glass of water 3 times a day. This balances hormones naturally. This remedy is very effective for PCOS and menopausal symptoms.

## LIFESTYLE

Aerobic exercise such as running, swimming or cycling for at least 40 minutes, 3 times a week, and stretching exercise such as yoga 2 to 3 times a week.

**Reduce stress**

Practice Pranayama, meditation, Anulom Vilom.

## DEEP SLEEP MARMA

As with male baldness, see above.

Head massage; press into the scalp with your fingertips to stimulate circulation.

## DIET

Follow the general hair loss diet as above.

## HERBS

**Ayushakti's Sukesha**, as above.

For hormonal imbalance you can also take **Ayushakti's Stree Sanjivani.**

# Alopecia Areata

Alopecia areata is a type of hair loss that occurs when your immune system mistakenly attacks your hair follicles. The damage to the follicle is usually not permanent. Typically, one or more bald patches appear on the scalp. These tend to be round and about the size of a large coin. Apart from the bald patch or patches, the scalp usually looks healthy and there is no scarring. Occasionally there may be mild redness, mild scaling, mild burning, or a slightly itchy feeling on the bald patches.

## Causes

Alopecia areata occurs most frequently in people who have family members with the condition. This suggests that heredity may be a causal factor. In addition, it is slightly more likely to occur in people who have relatives with autoimmune diseases. The condition is thought to be a systemic autoimmune disorder, in which the body attacks its own anagen hair follicles and suppresses or stops hair growth. For example, T-cell lymphocytes cluster around affected follicles, causing inflammation and subsequent hair loss.

### HOME REMEDY

| | |
|---|---|
| Pomegranate juice | ½ cup |
| Banana | 1 |
| Sweet grape juice | ½ cup |
| Amalaki (Emblica officinalis) powder | 1 tsp |
| Maka (Eclipta alba) powder | 1 tsp |

Make a smoothie of it all and drink at least twice a day

### LIFESTYLE AND EXERCISE

Yoga stretches and kapalbhati.

Deep sleep is necessary, see the Sleep section for advice.

## DIET

General hair loss diet as above.

## HERBS

**Ayushakti's Sukesha** (tablets) is most effective in dealing with hair loss.

To improve immunity you can also take **Ayushakti's Ojas** tablets.

*For Ayushakti supplements and clinics, see page iv.*

# 11. Relieving Common Digestive Disorders

Dyspepsia, also known as indigestion, is a condition of impaired digestion which usually describes a group of symptoms rather than one predominant symptom.

Functional indigestion (previously called non-ulcer dyspepsia)is indigestion without evidence of an organic disease that is likely to explain the symptoms. In the majority of cases indigestion is linked to eating and/or drinking habits. Sometimes it may be caused by infection or medication. Most people will experience some symptoms of indigestion in their lives.

Allopathic medicine is focused on organic damage and may overlook the function of the digestive tract. The gastrointestinal tract is a very integrated system via nervous and hormonal regulation, and all medications have side effects of disruption or turning off some of the digestive function. There is poor understanding of dyspepsia and consequently no specific care from standard medical treatment is given to tackle the problem from the root level.

## Common causes of dyspepsia

- Wrong eating habits: eating and drinking wrong things at wrong times and in wrong quantities.
- Emotional trauma, nervousness as stressful events produce responses in the gut.
- Smoking
- Gastritis (inflammation of the stomach), peptic ulcers, pancreatitis (inflammation of the pancreas), gall stones, hiatus hernia (weakening of valve between stomach and oesophagus).
- Infection, especially with bacteria known as Helicobacter pylori
- Some medications, such as antibiotics and NSAIDs (non-steroid anti-inflammatory drugs).

### AYURVEDIC POINT OF VIEW

All digestion is dependent upon proper functioning of the digestive fire or Agni. Ajirna or indigestion is caused by the vitiation of Agni. This is caused by the following:

- Eating too fast, over eating, or irregular eating.
- Intake of unwholesome, heavy, cold, un-unctuous, or contaminated food.
- Improper use of purgation, emetic, and oelation therapy.
- Living in improper country, or seasons.
- Suppression of natural urges which in turn creates Ama which is a undigested food converted into toxins.

# Abdominal Pain

Abdominal pain is pain that occurs between the chest and pelvic regions. Abdominal pain can be crampy, achy, dull, intermittent or sharp. It's also called a stomach ache. Inflammation or diseases that affect the organs in the abdomen can cause abdominal pain. Viral, bacterial, or parasitic infections that affect the stomach and intestines may also cause significant pain in abdomen.

It could also be because of menstrual cramps.

## HOME REMEDY

| | |
|---|---|
| Ajwain powder | 1 tsp |
| Jeera powder | ½ tsp |
| Dry ginger powder | ½ tsp |
| Hing | 4 pinches |

Mix all in 1 cup of warm water and drink twice a day.

## GENERAL DIET GUIDELINES FOR INDIGESTION

**To avoid:** Foods such as wheat, refined white flour, meat (especially red meat) and refined sugar decrease the digestive fire (Agni) and produce toxins (Ama). Deep fried food Beans and raw salads are heavy to digest and highly Vata (air) increasing or gas forming. Hot/spicy foods, alcohol, caffeine, smoking increases Pitta, acidity, and heat in body. Ice cold foods and drinks are immediate 'killers 'for the digestive fire. They also produce excess mucus.

**Foods to enjoy:** Eating small and regular meals and a healthy balanced diet is very important to beat all digestive health concerns. Cooked vegetables such as pumpkin (kaddu), squashes, marrow, courgette, spinach, fenugreek leaves (Methi), French beans, bottle gourd (Dudhi), ridge gourd (Turai), snake gourd (Padwal), smooth gourd (Galka), mange-tout, asparagus, fennel, swede, sweet corn, onion, carrots, parsnips beetroot, celery, chicory and leeks. However, potatoes should only be taken occasionally, with skin.

Pulses are an essential part of a healthy diet. Mung and split mung beans (green gram), tuvar dal (pigeon peas)and masoor dal (red lentils) are easy to digest, balancing and nourishing to the body. To get the full value from pulses they should be eaten together with grains (especially rice).

Grains including rice, oat, rye, maize (Makai), millets (Jawar, Bajra Nachani) amaranth (Rajigira), quinoa, kamut, spelt, polenta, basically everything other than wheat. Flours made from the above grains and also from potatoes and buckwheat are excellent substitutes for 'normal 'flour.

Dry fruits like almonds, walnuts, apricots, figs, hazel nuts, dates, raisins can be used.

One can enjoy white meat like chicken, turkey, fishes (river water) occasionally, if you are non vegetarian.

One can replace dairy milk by almond milk, rice milk, soya milk or oat milk.

## LIFESTYLE

- Avoid smoking and drinking alcohol.
- Avoid stress.

- Avoid eating too much, too fast and at wrong times.
- Eat on time, don't stay hungry for long.
- Take proper and timely sleep.
- Drink lukewarm (boiled) water throughout the day.
- Exercise daily, walking, swimming, dancing, and cycling are all good.
- Practise Yoga and Pranayama (Anulom, Vilom).
- Practice meditation to beat stress.

**AYUSHAKTI HERBAL REMEDIES**

**Gulkacid:** 1 tablet twice a day—digests Ama and pacifies excess Pitta and acidity

**Gasmukti:** 1 tablet twice a day—pacifies excess Vata/air in abdomen

## Bloating, gas, and distension

The most commonly recognized signs of indigestion are 'gas 'and heaviness, bloating and hence distension on tummy. Gas is universally looked upon as an embarrassment and many of us avoid foods like pulses and potato that produce gas. Gas is a natural by-product of digestion and metabolism, and every system produces a certain amount in the process of digestion. But in a healthy system gas either gets diluted, or dissolved and is eliminated from the body through the large intestine and other outlets. Some people complain that on eating certain foods, they get gas. But according to Ayurveda, that is the function of the those foods to stimulate the collection of isolated gas pockets and bring them all to the gas chamber - the stomach from where they can be more easily expelled. Each individual has his/her own unique constitution and is or is not able to digest certain foods accordingly.

Bloating can be described as the feeling that there is an inflated balloon in the abdomen. It is a commonly reported symptom and is sometimes associated with distension, or the visible increase in the width of the area between your hips and chest (abdominal girth).

Both bloating and distension cause discomfort, and sometimes pain, and have a negative impact on the quality of life for some individuals. The symptoms may be linked with other gas related complaints, such as burping or belching.

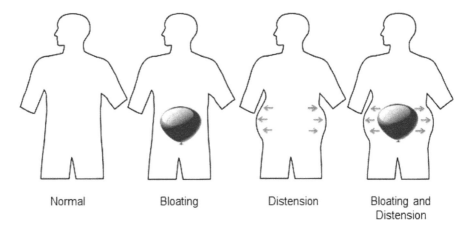

Normal          Bloating          Distension          Bloating and Distension

## Possible reasons for bloating and distension

- Too much gas in the intestine
- Abnormal levels of bacteria in the small intestine (small intestinal bacterial overgrowth – SIBO)
- Intolerance to certain foods

## DIET AND LIFESTYLE

As mentioned in Abdominal pain section.

## HOME REMEDIES FOR DISTENSION

**1.**

| | |
|---|---|
| Ajwain powder | 1 tsp |
| Dry ginger powder | ½ tsp |
| Hing (asafoetida) | 4 pinches |
| Black pepper | 4 pinches |
| Rock salt | 4 pinches |

Mix all in ½ cup of warm water and drink twice a day

**2.**

Take 1 tsp castor oil daily at night with warm water.

**3.**

Apply a paste of ¼ tsp of asafoetida and ¼ tsp of ajwain (carom seeds) powder around naval area.

### AYUSHAKTI HERBAL REMEDIES

**Supachak:** 2 tablets twice a day—improves digestion

**Gasmukti:** 1 tablet twice a day—pacifies excess gas

# Acidity/hyperacidity

Hyperacidity is a medical condition in which the stomach secretes a lot of acids. It can be caused due to various reasons.

Hyperacidity has various symptoms which can include:

- Sudden pain in stomach, burning pain
- Nausea and vomiting
- Loss of appetite
- Flatulence
- Heartburn

Sometimes, the problem aggravates and leads to other complications such as chronic indigestion and gastric ulcers.

In Ayurveda, Hyperacidity (Amlapitta) is also because of vitiation of Pitta dosha in stomach, resulting abnormally sour Pitta, it's also caused by increased digestive fire, which converts even food into excess acid.

So pacification of excess Pitta and increased Agni (digestive fire) is very important in treating acidity.

### Hyperacidity causes

- Helicobacter pylori infection (a specific bacteria in stomach cause severe, chronic acidity
- Hiatus hernia (weakening of stomach valve which causes acid reflux)
- Medications
- Alcohol
- Smoking
- Eating habits
- Stress

DIET AND LIFESTYLE

As under abdominal pain.


HOME REMEDIES FOR ACIDITY

**1.**

| | |
|---|---|
| Black raisins | 20, soaked in water and extracted into ½ glass water |
| Yastimadhu (liquorice) powder | ½ tsp |
| Amla powder (Emblica officinalis) | 1 tsp |
| Jeera (cumin seed) powder | ½ tsp |
| Variyali (fennel seed) powder | ½ tsp |
| Shunthi (ginger) powder | ¼ tsp |
| Elaichi (cardamom) powder | ¼ tsp |

Mix and drink this twice a day.

**2.**

Take 1 tsp ghee on an empty stomach in the morning.


AYUSHAKTI HERBAL REMEDIES

**Gulkacid**: 2 tablets twice a day—pacifies Pitta and specially act of helicobacter pylori, acidity, heartburn, gastritis, and acid reflux

For chronic symptoms, you can take 2 tablets 4 times a day.

# Diarrhoea

It is the condition of having at least three loose or liquid bowel movements each day. It often lasts for a few days and can result in dehydration due to fluid loss. Diarrhoea is the body's natural defence mechanism against a harmful virus or bacterium, an ingested toxin, or a food that disagrees with the digestive system. Diarrhoea the most common cause is an infection of the intestines due to either a virus bacteria or parasite; a condition known as gastroenteritis. These infections are often acquired from food or water that has been contaminated by stool, or directly from another person who is infected.

It may be divided into three types:

- short duration watery diarrhoea
- short duration bloody diarrhoea
-  if it lasts for more than two weeks, persistent diarrhoea.

If blood is present it is also known as dysentery.

The number of non-infectious causes may include:

- hyperthyroidism
- lactose intolerance
- inflammatory bowel disease (ulcerative colitis, chrohn's disease, celiac disease)
- irritable bowel syndrome (IBS)
- number of medications

According to Ayurveda, diarrhoea occurs when the digestive fire is weakened, usually by excess Pitta. Absorption and assimilation slow, and the movement of food through the digestive system is accelerated – causing liquid stools. The remedy is to pacify Pitta and to gently kindle Agni.

LIFESTYLE AND DIET

As described. Proper sanitation and pure drinking water.

**HOME REMEDIES**

**1.**

| | |
|---|---|
| Dry ginger powder (sunthi) | ¼ tsp |
| Cumin seed powder (jeera) | 1 tsp |
| Poppy seed paste | ¼ tsp |
| Salt | 1 pinch |
| Fresh curds | 1 tblsp |

Mix well and take twice a day.

**2.**

Drink pomegranate juice twice a day.
Peel half a pomegranate; add 2 cups of water.

**3.**

| | |
|---|---|
| Cooked rice | 1 cup |
| Ghee | ½ tsp |
| Dry ginger (sunthi) powder | ¼ tsp |
| Cumin (jeera) powder | ½ tsp |
| Fresh curds | 3 to 4 tblsp |

Mix well and eat.

## AYUSHAKTI HERBAL REMEDIES

**Aampachak**: 1 tablet twice a day—improves digestive fire, reduces inflammation

**Dyromukti**: 1 tablet twice a day—stop diarrhoea instantly and reduces inflammation.

If you have IBS (irritable bowel syndrome) then you need to take this herb for a year or two. You will find relief in 2 to 3 months.

# Ulcerative Colitis

## HOME REMEDIES

For ulcerative colitis with bleeding

| | |
|---|---|
| Curds | 200 g |
| Cardamom powder | ¼ tsp |
| Nutmeg | 1 pinch |

Pour the curds on a piece of muslin and leave it to strain for one hour. Discard the water and mix the curds with the other ingredients. In serious cases, drink it two to three times a day after meals. The diarrhoea and bleeding will naturally cease in about two or three days.

# Nausea

Also called as motion sickness or feeling sick. This is a sensation of unease and discomfort in the upper stomach with an involuntary urge to vomit. Generally a stomach illness or pregnancy can cause nausea, other causes may include:

- Medication induced
- Gall bladder disease
- Food poisoning
- Infections
- Overeating
- Ulcers

Nausea often is associated with headaches, dizziness, vomiting, abdominal pain, heart burn.

### AYURVEDA PERSPECTIVE

When digestive fire becomes weakened usually by derangement of Pachak Pitta, food remains undigested, which leads to formation of Ama.

### LIFESTYLE AND DIET CHANGES

As per section 1.

Advice: do not over-eat, eat on time.

## HOME REMEDY

½ tsp dry ginger powder + ¼ tsp rock salt drink with warm water before meals.

10 to 12 black raisins soaked overnight take empty stomach in morning.

## AYUSHAKTI HERBAL REMEDIES

**Gulkacid**: 2 tablets twice a day—pacifies Pitta, acidity

**Supachak**: 1 tablet twice a day—improves digestion

**Amrutras**: 1 tablet twice a day—pacifies Pitta, digests Ama, and reduces motion sickness

# Constipation

Constipation can be defined as:

- infrequent bowel movements (typically three times or fewer per week)
- difficulty during defecation (straining during more than 25% of bowel movements or a subjective sensation of hard stools)
- the sensation of incomplete bowel evacuation.

Some common causes of constipation include:

- Antacid medicines containing calcium or aluminium
- Changes in your usual diet or activities
- Colon cancer
- Eating a lot of dairy products
- Eating disorders

- Irritable bowel syndrome (IBS)
- Neurological conditions such as Parkinson's disease or multiple sclerosis
- Not being active
- Not enough water or fibre in your diet
- Overuse of laxatives (over time, this weakens the bowel muscles)
- Pregnancy
- Problems with the nerves and muscles in the digestive system
- Resisting the urge to have a bowel movement, which some people do because of haemorrhoids
- Some medications (especially strong pain drugs such as narcotics, antidepressants, or iron pills)
- Stress
- Underactive thyroid (hypothyroidism)

According to Ayurveda, it is usually a Vata disorder, particularly if it is a long-standing condition or in the elderly. It may also be due to high Pitta (heat which dries out the stool) or high Kapha (mucous congestion clogging the colon).

Proper assimilation of food and elimination of faeces are important for maintaining health. Improper elimination from the colon causes retention of waste and morbid matter, which results in systemic poisoning or autointoxication. When the colon does not function promptly, the result is an accumulation of offensive and highly poisonous wastes; Ayurveda calls it 'Ama'. Ama is considered as root cause of most of the ailments as per Ayurveda.

The normal duration between the times the food is eaten until the faeces is expelled, is normally between 16 to 24 hours. If the residue remains for more than 24 hrs, it gives rise to toxins.

## LIFESTYLE AND DIET

As per mentioned earlier.

## HOME REMEDIES

1 cup warm milk with 1 tsp of ghee at night.

10 black raisins soaked overnight to take in morning.

Figs (Anjeer): boil a few figs in a glass of milk, drink this mixture at night before bed. Make sure the mixture is warm when you drink it.

Flax seeds (Alsi): 2 tsp of flax seeds powder with warm water on empty stomach in morning.

## AYUSHAKTI HERBAL REMEDIES

**Aampachak**: 1 tablet twice a day—improves digestion and eliminates mucus

**Amrutadi churna**: 1 to 2 teaspoons at night—improves digestion and herbal laxative

# Loss of Appetite

Many possible causes exist for a decreased appetite, some of which may be harmless, while others indicate a serious clinical condition or pose a significant risk. Loss of appetite causes unintentional weight loss.

Common factors responsible for loss of appetite:

- Depression, sadness, grief, anxiety
- Digestive problems such as pain in abdomen, hyperacidity,
- Anorexia nervosa
- Acute viral hepatitis
- Cancer, AIDS
- Chronic kidney disease

## AN AYURVEDIC PERSPECTIVE

Loss of appetite and indigestion are closely linked aspects of digestive disturbance in Ayurveda. *Agnimandhya*is the term used to denote loss of appetite while *Ajeerna* denotes indigestion. A harmonious balance of *Vata* and *Pitta* describes the essence of a normal appetite. A vitiation in their mutual balance could lead to a loss of appetite. Irregular dietary habits bring about a vitiation in *Pitta* while psychic problems like anxiety, fear or physical causes like suppression of impeding urges lead to an imbalance in *Vata*. Both these sequences lead to disturbances in normal levels of appetite.

## DIET AND LIFESTYLE

As described earlier.

## Suggested ways of improving the appetite are as follows:

- Set times of the day when you are normally hungry. Eat at those times even if you do not feel particularly hungry.
- Eat small meals 5-6 times a day.

- Eat protein-rich foods.
- Drink nutritious fluids (such as milk or juice) between meals instead of during meals. Drinking too much during a meal can make you feel full too quickly.
- Take a 20 minute walk about an hour before eating.
- Light exercise helps stimulate appetite.
- Avoid distractions, such as the television, while serving meals.
- Keep the table simple. Place only the food and utensils on the table.
- Make sure the food is at the right temperature.
- Serve only one or two dishes at a time.
- Allow ample time to eat.
- Family members should eat together.

## HOME REMEDY

**1.**

1 cup pomegranate juice + ¼ tsp rock salt + 1 tsp honey.

Take daily on an empty stomach, in the morning.

**2.**

1 teaspoon of amla powder with ½ teaspoon rock salt before meals increases appetite.

**3.**

Mix in equal parts each ½ teaspoon of cinnamon bark, small cardamom, coriander seeds and fennel seeds. Soak the mixture in cold water overnight. Strain this blend with a tea strainer. Drinking this cold infusion early in the morning helps in building an appetite.

## AYUSHAKTI HERBAL REMEDIES

**Supachak**: 2 tablets twice a day—improves digestion, reduces bloating, fullness

**Livtone**: 2 tablets twice a day—increases appetite

**Sumedha**: 1 tablet twice a day—for anxiety and depression

*For Ayushakti supplements and clinics, see page iv.*

# Diet, Health and the Stages of Life

If you would like to live a good long life, but remain full of good health, vitality, and mental and physical stamina, it's important to follow healthy habits on a daily basis. It's not so good to wait for a health problem to occur and then fix it. This way of working is in fact waiting for the body to revolt against the mistreatment of years, when all of a sudden you get a big shock, wake up and then start to work on your health.

What is necessary is that you have to work on your health on a daily basis, watching out every day for the little signals that tell us what to do, and make sure you find balance every day of your life.

This means that it's very important that you follow certain daily routines that lead to an energised daily life. This routine has to include using certain kinds of marma points; and a diet and exercise programme which constantly improves your circulation, to keep your Agni high and lead to having great, deep sleep, so that you wake up in the morning completely rested and fresh.

During the day eat the right foods, so that you are completely aware and alert when you are working rather than feeling tired. Good food also digests well, so it doesn't create Ama, toxic mucus.

At the same time, life is for living fully in every moment, and about being in balance, so I will tell you how to design your own diet, what kind of daily routine one has to follow so that every day you are taking care of your health, little by little, even if you have no problems, you will avoid problems.

Sometimes when you slip out of your careful routine and eat something wrong, you can learn how to restore balance, because life is about enjoyment. Enjoy all the kinds of food that you love, but learn how to clear toxins immediately after eating something which is not so good, and restore essential balance.

## The stages of life according to age

## Kapha—stage one

It is important to understand the effect of the different stages of our lives, so that we can take them into account in the way we live and eat. Until the age of 15, we often get coughs, which is a natural consequence of it being the Kapha time of life. So when children get coughs and colds, don't just react and give antibiotics or other medication from the doctor's. Simply stop giving him or her milk and wheat, and you will see a magical change within two days; the condition will diminish dramatically.

I'll share with you the example of my own son. By the time he was five months old he had asthma. Because his father also had asthma, he was probably born with this allergy. One day he just lay there without moving, and I was a bit shocked. Sometimes I am a mother rather than a doctor, so I panicked and I thought; Oh, God, what's happening?

My mother brain didn't allow my doctor brain to work, so I got a paediatric friend to come and check him out. She said he is suffering from breathlessness and severe wheezing, and that he would have to use inhalers, at least until he was 10 or 12 years old.

When she left I thought this; if I give an inhaler to my son, I have no right to treat anybody else's son on this planet as an Ayurvedic doctor; I won't do this because I know that Ayurveda works. So I gave him three Ayushakti formulas to enhance his immune system: Asthaloc, D-Vyro, and Kaphno syrup to improve respiratory function.

I gave these formulas to him for one and a half years, and kept him off milk and wheat products for two to three years. When I tell this to mothers, they say, 'Oh, what can I give them to eat? 'The truth is that there is a huge variety of food available these days, like oatmeal and almond milk, spelt bread, pasta without wheat, and so on, so it's quite possible to eat normal food without milk or wheat; there's always an alternative.

My son is now 16 years old and has had no breathlessness attacks since he was a baby. And he understands his allergy issue so well that he now monitors himself. Whenever he gets a cough (which is not so often), he stops eating milk products and wheat, and gets 50 per cent better in two days. He puts lots of black pepper on his food, sometimes a bit of chilli, and this too makes a real difference in reducing mucus. Apart from this he eats everything. In this way we have our health in our own hands; reduce mucus-enhancing foods and eat spicy foods; it's really simple.

As soon as your cough has gone you can return to your normal diet and you'll be fine, because your body is now ready to take it. But if you think that you can have milk when you have a cough or cold, you're mistaken; this would overload your system, you'd only make things worse. Since their metabolism is very active, children should eat five portions a day with one portion of fried or oily food. Most children can digest heavy food, wheat, and so on, at this age.

## Pitta—stage two

It's the same with Pitta. Between the ages of 15 and 40, Pitta, and its natural heat, runs high. This may lead to headaches. High acidity, and skin problems such as acne. So, during this period, make sure that you don't eat a lot of spicy foods, sour or fermented foods such tomatoes, lemons, vinegar, alcohol, anything which is fermented. There are always alternatives, such as using limes instead of lemons, for example.

These sour and fermented foods produce acidity, headaches, acne, and skin problems, so whenever these things trouble you, stay away from them. If headaches, skin problems or acidity are chronic problems for you, it's best to stay away from them for several months, until the problem has been handled. This is what is known as balancing. When Pitta is high, the appetite is good and you can eat large portions. You can digest even fried food and can handle a moderate amount of wheat.

For most people, our body has high level of Pitta roughly between the ages of 15 and 40. This means that between those ages we can do lots of things, we can achieve a lot. After 40 this Pitta energy diminishes in our brains and bodies, in a natural way, and because of that, our ambition, our power to achieve, gradually diminishes.

So the wise thing is to work hard and smart between the ages of 20 and 40, do your best to achieve what you can, and keep aside some finances from this period for the time when your body is going to work a little bit less actively than before.

## Vata—stage three

After 40 or 45 there comes a time of what we call diminishing, when aging comes on slowly, step by step, and at that time of life it's natural that you have higher Vata. People who have high Vata by nature may develop extreme Vata, which can cause osteoporosis, or osteoarthritis, sometimes by the age of 45.

This means that after that age you have to take care of Vata related issues. You should always be careful with what you eat; it should always be liquid, soupy, predominantly vegetables. Balancing Vata is vital after the age of 45, so food should be cooked, which means fewer foods such as raw vegetables that increase the production of gas, which leads to an increase in Vata.

After 40, when our metabolism slows down, I advise people to cut down on wheat, fried food, and red meat from that age. After 40, the key is to reduce carbohydrates, eat lots of soupy cooked food with vegetables, mung, and lentils.

## Ama, allergies, wheat and meat

These days even children are allergic to wheat; it takes a long time to digest, which is OK for children as they are constantly running round and moving, but we don't do this so much when we are grown up. This means that after the age of fifteen it's better to either cut down on or stop wheat and red meat completely. Another food we must take care with is yoghurt. I believe, and Ayurveda says, that it blocks our channels, and you must stay away from anything that does this. It's OK to eat yoghurt now and again, when you feel like it, but not as a daily habit.

As wheat and red meat produce a huge amount of channel-blocking Ama, stay away from them as much as possible, and after the age of 40 stop eating them completely. My teacher, who lived to be 124 years old, and other people who live very, very long and healthy lives, with healthy minds and active bodies—from my research—stopped eating wheat, red meat and deep fried food from the age of 40 or 50.

The truth is that we can't process wheat and heavy foods well after the age of 40 or 50, so we need to stay away from them. If you do get tempted to eat them, or occasionally eat junk food, ending up with heaviness in your stomach, just restrict yourself the next day to vegetables and mung soup. This is a kind of fasting; eating the opposite to the heavy food that caused a problem.

It's the same principle as turning on the air-conditioner when you feel hot, or the heater when you feel cold; with our bodies; when you feel heavy, eat simple food, something that makes you feel light like warm mung bean soup, which is fantastic.

## Raw food, digestion and the stages of life

We all love raw food, and people say that it is full of living energy that is very good for you. I agree with this, but around 80 per cent of vitamins and minerals are not destroyed by cooking, they can take the heat, and when cooked are far more digestible.

If you go to an extreme and eat only raw food it will lead to acidity, because it doesn't all get digested and what remains ferments. I've seen people blending fruit and greens and vegetables and just drinking that as their only food. In a few months, or even weeks, they can develop acidity and colitis, because not so many people can digest this kind of food well.

Greens such as spinach and arugula (rocket) are fine, because their raw fibres can be digested, but fibres from the skin of fruit, and heavy vegetables like carrots and beets, are difficult to digest. They have to be cooked so that these fibres, which help reduce cholesterol naturally, are easily absorbed.

When people are young, say under 15, they can eat lots of fat, so I tell people to give lots of cheese and milk and meat, fatty things, to their children—if they aren't allergic to these things.

However, between 15 and 40, our metabolism diminishes and the hormones change in both women and men. At that time it's important to reduce wheat, deep fried foods and red meat, as much as possible. Children and grown-ups should eat in opposite proportions.

This means that the diet of young children, who need lots of carbohydrates and protein, can be 30% vegetables, 30% proteins, 30% carbohydrates and 10% fats. Between the ages of 15 and 40 you should increase your vegetable intake to 50% of your diet, with protein at 30%, and 20% carbohydrates. Carbohydrates include rice, potatoes, all cereals, fruit and a little sugar. Protein means eggs, all the dals and lentils and fish and chicken—and, of course, red meat. I always tell people not to eat red meat after the age of 25, because this leads to arteries getting clogged, blockages in the heart and high cholesterol. This means that you have to start taking care with your diet by the age 25 or 30 if you don't want to get heart problems in the future.

Then, after the age of 40 or 45, in order to remain fit and healthy and free from cholesterol, arthritis, heart problems, high uric acid and other health problems that come at that age, make sure that you eat only 10% or 20% carbohydrates—two or three spoonfuls of rice, or half a slice of bread—and 20% protein, with 60 to 70% of the meal being cooked vegetables or a little salad, or a mixture of both.

## Smita's story of changing metabolism

To give you an example, I'd like to share my own story. I used to always be fantastically fit and skinny; weighing 53 kilos, which is perfect for my height of 5'4'. When I became pregnant I practised yoga and followed a perfect Ayurvedic regimen with herbs and other practices, for the full term of my pregnancy. When my boy was born, because of those practices, my weight went down from 66 kilos back to 54 kilos in just in 10 days.

I continued to maintain that weight, but as soon as I reached 45 something changed. My hormones completely changed, my emotions changed; I felt irritable, less calm, less tolerant and my body bloated greatly. I would regularly put on one kilo or more every month.

In spite of the heavy exercise—yoga, running, and swimming—that I've been doing for 30 years, I continued to put on a kilo every month. At that time I realised that I needed to take natural herbs that I hadn't taken before, because I never needed them. I was managing my weight and health through my lifestyle and diet alone.

When I started taking natural herbs to balance my emotions, and specifically my hormones and metabolism, I felt an immediate shift, and changed my diet straight away. I cut down my wheat intake completely. Carbohydrates were around 20 per cent of my diet when I was 45, but now I am over 50 I can tolerate only 10 per cent. I bloat up straight away if I eat more than that.

I brought my weight back down again, to 54 kilos, just by taking herbs, along with my diet and daily exercise. The point is that life is about understanding where you are with yourself. When you take herbs, or follow a diet it doesn't mean that you are sick, it means that you are actually alert enough to prevent illness and take care of yourself; you control your own health.

Living like this makes such a powerful difference that major health problems such as diabetes, high cholesterol and high, blood pressure, everything will come nowhere near you, they'll find a door in someone else. Your body is not available, the door is closed to such things.

When you take this wisdom into account, and act according to your age and your needs, adapt your lifestyle, diet and so on, it means your health is in your hands.

# Index

Lightning Source UK Ltd.
Milton Keynes UK
UKHW031230131120
373344UK00006B/449